Pathophysiology

made

Incredibly

Visual! ™

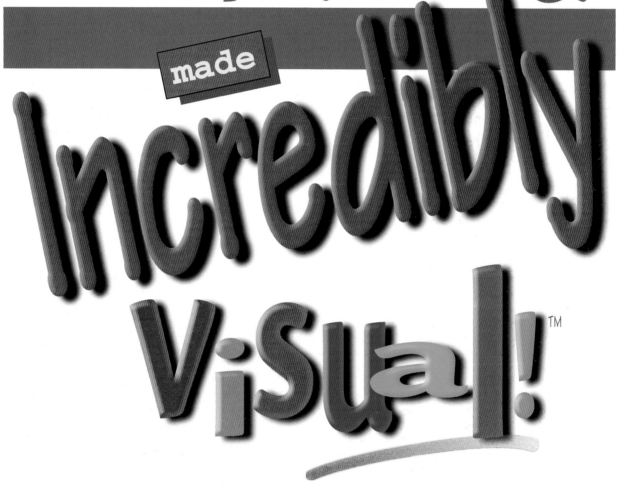

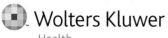 Wolters Kluwer | Lippincott Williams & Wilkins
Health

Philadelphia · Baltimore · New York · London
Buenos Aires · Hong Kong · Sydney · Tokyo

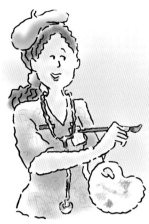

Staff

Executive Publisher
Judith A. Schilling McCann, RN, MSN

Editorial Director
David Moreau

Clinical Director
Joan M. Robinson, RN, MSN

Art Director
Mary Ludwicki

Senior Managing Editor
Tracy S. Diehl

Clinical Project Manager
Beverly Ann Tscheschlog, RN, BS

Editors
Karen C. Comerford, Brenna H. Mayer

Copy Editors
Kimberly Bilotta (supervisor), Amy Furman,
Shana Harrington, Dorothy P. Terry,
Pamela Wingrod

Designer
Lynn Foulk

Illustrators
Bot Roda, Esteban Cabrera, Judy Newhouse,
Leah Rhoades Purvis, Betty Winnberg

Digital Composition Services
Diane Paluba (manager), Joyce Rossi Biletz,
Donna S. Morris

Associate Manufacturing Manager
Beth J. Welsh

Editorial Assistants
Megan L. Aldinger, Karen J. Kirk, Linda K. Ruhf

Design Assistant
Georg W. Purvis IV

Indexer
Barbara Hodgson

The clinical treatments described and recommended in this publication are based on research and consultation with nursing, medical, and legal authorities. To the best of our knowledge, these procedures reflect currently accepted practice. Nevertheless, they can't be considered absolute and universal recommendations. For individual applications, all recommendations must be considered in light of the patient's clinical condition and, before administration of new or infrequently used drugs, in light of the latest package-insert information. The authors and publisher disclaim any responsibility for any adverse effects resulting from the suggested procedures, from any undetected errors, or from the reader's misunderstanding of the text.

Printed in China.

PIV010307

Library of Congress Cataloging-in-Publication Data
Pathophysiology made incredibly visual.
   p. ; cm.
   Includes bibliographical references and index.
   1. Physiology, Pathological. 2. Physiology, Pathological — Atlases. I. Lippincott Williams & Wilkins.
   [DNLM: 1. Disease. 2. Pathology. 3. Physiology. QZ 140 P2943 2008]
RB113.P3637 2008
   616.07 — dc22
ISBN-13: 978-1-58255-555-3 (alk. paper)
ISBN-10: 1-58255-555-9 (alk. paper) 2006100518

Contents

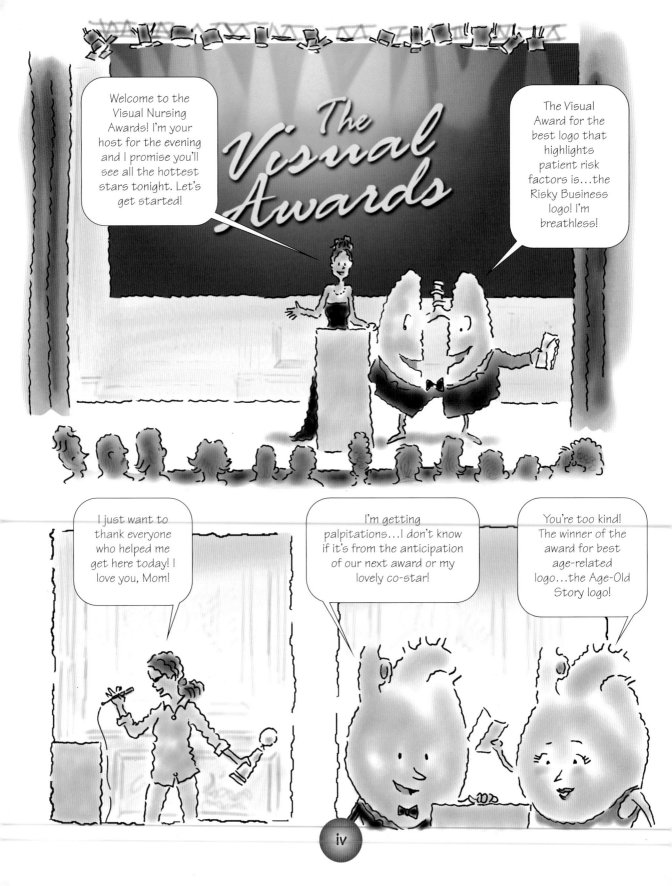

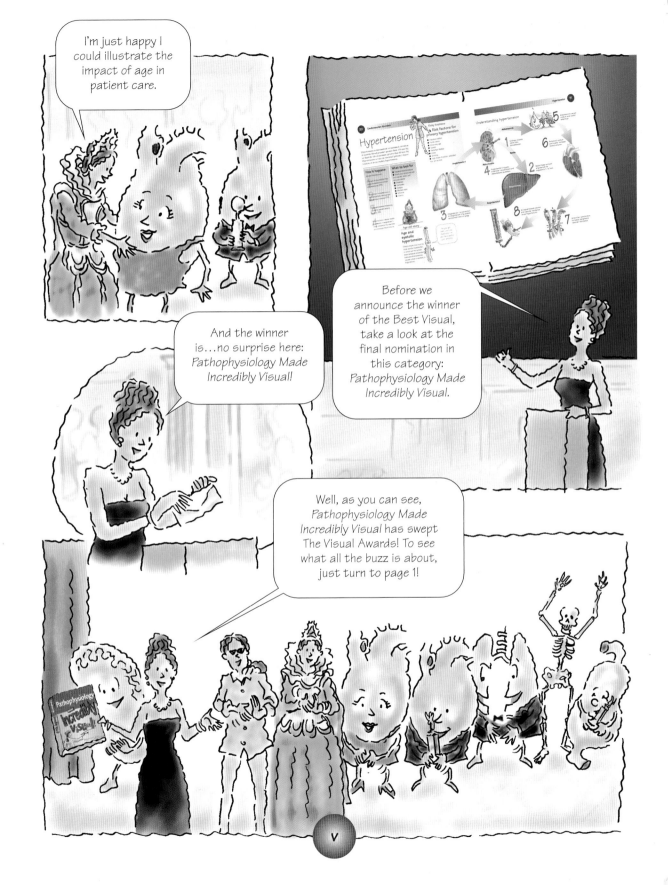

Contributors and consultants

Beverly Anderson, RN, MSN, MOT
Associate Professor
Malcolm X College
Chicago

Kim Cooper, RN, MSN
Nursing Department Chair
Ivy Tech Community College
Terre Haute, Ind.

Lillian Craig, RN, MSN, FNP-C
Adjunct Faculty
Oklahoma Panhandle State University
Goodwell

Michelle Helderman, RN, MSN
Nursing Instructor
Ivy Tech Community College
Terre Haute, Ind.

Bridget A. Howard, MSN, APRN,BC
Nurse Practitioner
Midwest Gastroenterology
Lee's Summit, Mo.

Theresa A. Petersen, RN, MSN
Assistant Professor
Montana State University – Northern
Havre

Monica Narvaez Ramirez, RN, MSN
Nursing Instructor
University of the Incarnate Word School
  of Nursing & Health Professions
San Antonio, Tex.

Ruthie Robinson, PhD, RN, FAEN, CCRN, CEN
Director, Center for Nursing Innovation
Christus Hospital
Beaumont, Tex.

MaryClare A. Schafer, RN, MS, ONC, CRRN
Director of Nursing
Rehabilitation Hospital of South Jersey
Vineland

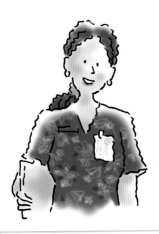

1
The basics

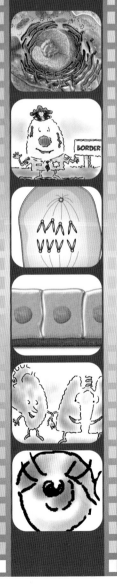

Cell basics...
cell division...
cell adaptation?
It all makes me
vant to return to
my cell, er, coffin.

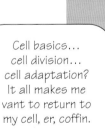

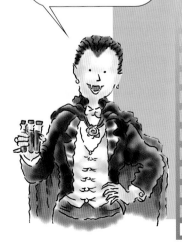

Cell basics

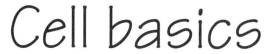

Just your average cell

The cell is the body's basic building block and the smallest living component of an organism. The human body consists of millions of cells grouped into highly specialized units that function together throughout the organism's life.

Large groups of individual cells form tissues, such as muscle, blood, and bone.

Tissues form the organs (such as the brain, heart, and liver), which are integrated into body systems (such as the central nervous system [CNS], cardiovascular system, and digestive system).

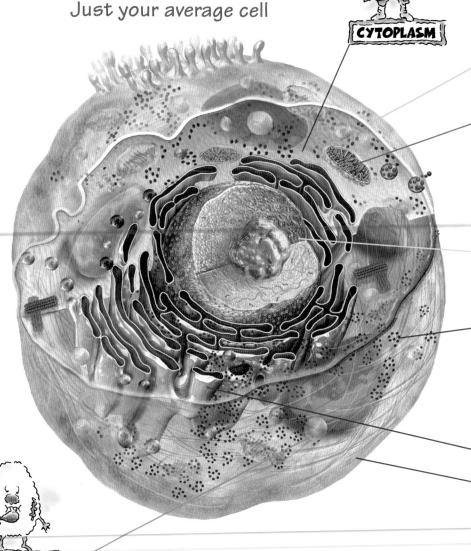

I surround and protect the nucleus.

CYTOPLASM

I'm the cell's digestive system.

LYSOSOME

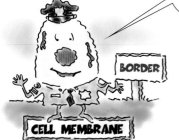

I'm the boundary system for the cell and I make sure that nothing escapes me!

BORDER

CELL MEMBRANE

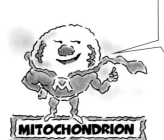

I'm the Mighty Mitochondrion and I give the cell energy.

MITOCHONDRION

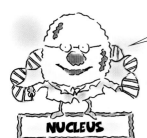

I'm the brain or control center of the cell. I carry most of the genetic material, so if you have red hair, it's probably because of me!

NUCLEUS

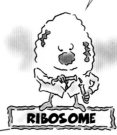

I combine protein and other material the cell needs.

RIBOSOME

I hold enzyme systems and I assist in the cell's metabolism.

GOLGI APPARATUS

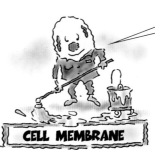

I protect the cell and transport material in and out of the cell. I am also the maintenance man for the cell's electrical activities that power cell function.

CELL MEMBRANE

Cell division

Before division, a cell must double its mass and content. This occurs during the growth phase, called *interphase*. Chromatin, the small, slender rods of the nucleus that give it its granular appearance, begins to form.

 Replication and duplication of deoxyribonucleic acid occurs during the four phases of mitosis.

The great divide

2 Metaphase

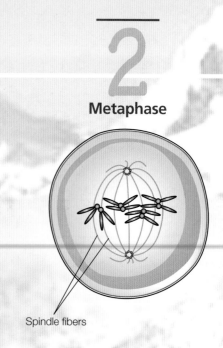

Spindle fibers

During metaphase, the centromeres divide, pulling the chromosomes apart. The centromeres then align themselves in the middle of the spindle.

1 Prophase

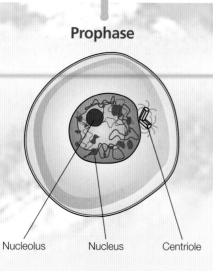

Nucleolus   Nucleus   Centriole

During prophase, the chromosomes coil and shorten, and the nuclear membrane dissolves. Each chromosome is made up of a pair of strands called *chromatids,* which are connected by a spindle of fibers called a *centromere.*

4
Telophase

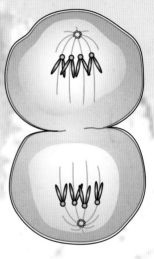

In the final phase of mitosis—telophase—a new membrane forms around each set of 46 chromosomes. The spindle fibers disappear, cytokinesis occurs, and the cytoplasm divides, producing two identical new daughter cells.

3
Anaphase

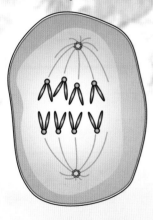

At the onset of anaphase, the centromeres begin to separate and pull the newly replicated chromosomes toward opposite sides of the cell. By the end of anaphase, 46 chromosomes are present on each side of the cell.

I wouldn't exactly say this is a "great" divide...

Cell adaptation

The cell faces many challenges through its life span. Stressors, changes in the body's health, disease, and other extrinsic and intrinsic factors can alter the cell's normal functioning.

Cells generally continue to function despite changing conditions or stressors. However, severe or prolonged stress or changes may injure or even destroy cells. When cell integrity is threatened, the cell reacts by drawing on its reserves to keep functioning by adaptive changes or by cellular dysfunction. If the cell's reserves are insufficient, the cell dies. If enough cellular reserve is available and the body doesn't detect abnormalities, the cell adapts by atrophy, hypertrophy, hyperplasia, metaplasia, or dysplasia.

Adaptive cell changes

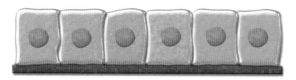

Normal cells

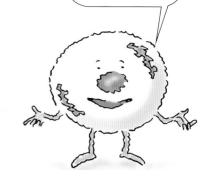

I guess you'd say I'm just your average cell.

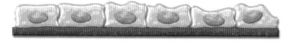

Atrophy

Atrophy is a reversible reduction in the size of the cell. It occurs as a result of disuse, insufficient blood flow, malnutrition, denervation, or reduced endocrine stimulation.

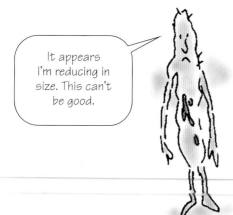

It appears I'm reducing in size. This can't be good.

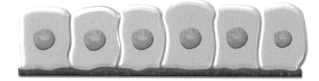

Hypertrophy

Hypertrophy is an enlargement of a cell due to an increased workload. It can result from normal physiologic conditions or abnormal pathologic conditions.

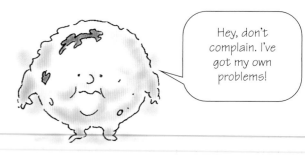

Hey, don't complain. I've got my own problems!

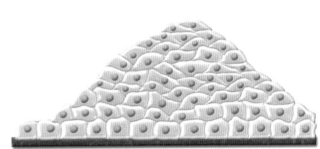

Hyperplasia

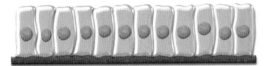

Hyperplasia is an increase in the number of cells caused by increased workload, hormonal stimulation, or decreased tissue.

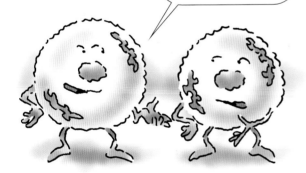

Metaplasia

Metaplasia is the replacement of one adult cell with another adult cell that can better endure the change or stress. It's usually a response to chronic inflammation or irritation.

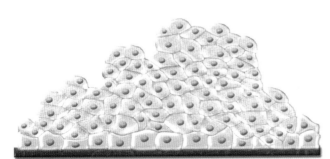

Dysplasia

In dysplasia, deranged cell growth of specific tissue results in abnormal size, shape, and appearance. Although dysplastic cell changes are adaptive and potentially reversible, they can precede cancerous changes.

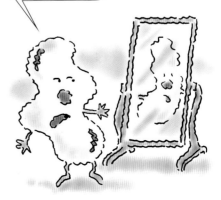

Cell injury

Injury to components of cells can lead to disease as the cells lose their ability to adapt. Cell injury may result from any of several intrinsic or extrinsic causes and may be classified as toxic, infectious, physical, or deficit.

memory board

To remember the four causes of cell injury, think of how the injury tipped (or *TIPD*) the scale of homeostasis:

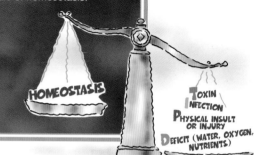

Toxic injury

Toxic injuries may be caused by factors inside the body (endogenous factors) or outside the body (exogenous factors). Common endogenous factors include genetically determined metabolic errors, gross malformations, and hypersensitivity reactions. Exogenous factors include alcohol, lead, carbon monoxide, and drugs that alter cellular function, such as chemotherapeutic agents or immunosuppressive drugs.

Deficit injury

When a deficit of water, oxygen, or nutrients occurs or if constant temperature and adequate waste disposal aren't maintained, cellular synthesis can't take place. A lack of just one of these basic requirements can cause cell disruption or death.

Infectious injury

Viral, fungal, protozoal, and bacterial organisms can cause cell injury or death. These organisms affect cell integrity, usually by interfering with cell synthesis, producing mutant cells. For example, human immunodeficiency virus alters the cell when the virus is replicated in the cell's ribonucleic acid.

Physical injury

Physical injury results from a disruption in the cell or in the relationships of the intracellular organelles (such as mitochondria, nuclei, lysosomes, and ribosomes). Two major types of physical injury are thermal (electrical or radiation) and mechanical (trauma or surgery).

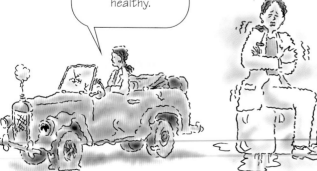

I hate to give you up, but I think it's time. Your carbon monoxide emissions are way beyond healthy.

Brrr! Frostbite can d-d-damage cells and cause ph-ph-physical injury and p-p-pain.

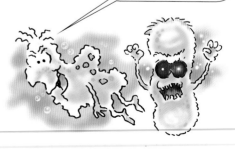

We can do a lot of damage by interfering with cell synthesis, producing mutant cells.

Stress and disease

When a stressor such as a life change occurs, a person can respond in one of two ways—by adapting successfully or by failing to adapt. A maladaptive response to stress may result in disease. The underlying stressor may be real or perceived.

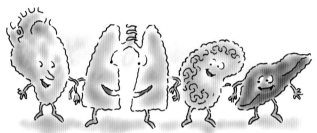

Hans Selye, a pioneer in the study of stress and disease, described stages of adaptation to a stressful event: alarm, resistance, and exhaustion or recovery. The stress response is controlled by actions taking place in the nervous and endocrine systems. These actions try to redirect energy to the organ—such as the heart, lungs, or brain—that's most affected by the stress.

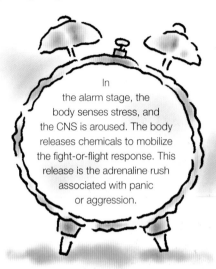

In the alarm stage, the body senses stress, and the CNS is aroused. The body releases chemicals to mobilize the fight-or-flight response. This release is the adrenaline rush associated with panic or aggression.

When stress strikes

According to Hans Selye's General Adaptation Model, the body reacts to stress in the stages depicted here.

Physical or psychological stressor

Alarm reaction
■ Arousal of the CNS begins. ■ Epinephrine and norepinephrine, along with other hormones, are released, causing an increase in heart rate, oxygen intake, and mental activity and increased force of heart contractions.

Resistance
■ The body responds to the stressor and attempts to return to homeostasis. ■ Coping mechanisms, such as avoidance or sublimation, are used.

Recovery	Exhaustion
	■ The body can no longer produce hormones such as in the alarm stage. ■ Organ damage begins.

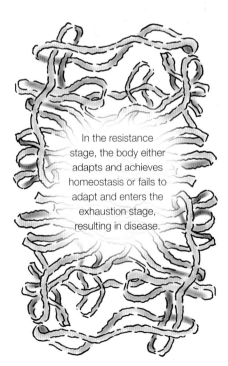

In the resistance stage, the body either adapts and achieves homeostasis or fails to adapt and enters the exhaustion stage, resulting in disease.

VISION QUEST

Able to label?

Label the parts of a cell indicated in this illustration.

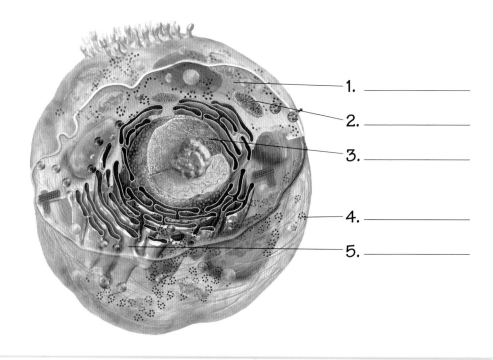

1. _____
2. _____
3. _____
4. _____
5. _____

Show and tell

Identify the four phases of mitosis shown in these illustrations and explain what happens in each phase.

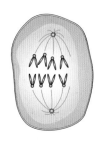 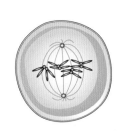 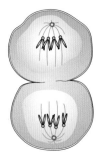 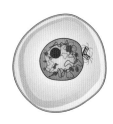

1. _____
2. _____
3. _____
4. _____
_____

2
Cardiovascular disorders

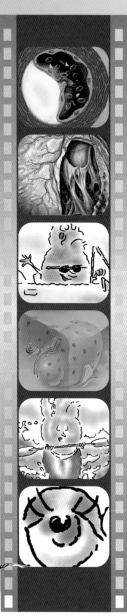

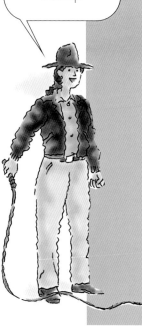

In my line of work, you can't afford heart problems. I'm sure this chapter will help everyone learn how heart problems develop.

Acute coronary syndromes

Acute myocardial infarction (MI), including ST-segment elevation MI and non-ST-segment elevation MI, and unstable angina are part of a group of diseases called *acute coronary syndromes* (ACSs).

How it happens

Plaque in the coronary arteries ruptures or erodes.

Platelets adhere to damaged area and become exposed to activating factors (collagen, thrombin, von Willebrand's factor).

Platelet activation produces glycoprotein IIb and IIIa receptors that bind fibrinogen.

Platelet aggregation and adhesion continue, enlarging the thrombus.

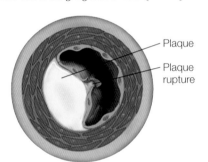

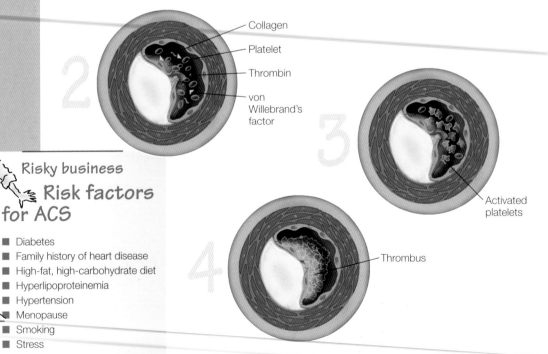

Plaque

Plaque rupture

Collagen

Platelet

Thrombin

von Willebrand's factor

Activated platelets

Thrombus

Risky business
Risk factors for ACS

- Diabetes
- Family history of heart disease
- High-fat, high-carbohydrate diet
- Hyperlipoproteinemia
- Hypertension
- Menopause
- Smoking
- Stress

What to look for

MI

- Chest pain (severe, persistent, squeezing, or crushing)
  - Usually in substernal chest
  - May radiate to left arm, neck, jaw, or shoulder blade
  - Unrelieved by rest or nitroglycerin
- Perspiration
- Anxiety
- Hypertension
- Feeling of impending doom
- Fatigue
- Shortness of breath
- Hypotension
- Nausea and vomiting

Unstable angina

- Chest pain (burning, squeezing, or crushing)
  - Usually in substernal or precordial chest
  - May radiate to left arm, neck, jaw, or shoulder blade
  - Relieved by nitroglycerin

Atypical chest pain

Women may experience chest pain typically associated with acute ischemia and MI; however, women—and occasionally men, elderly patients, and patients with diabetes—may also experience atypical chest pain. Signs and symptoms of atypical chest pain include:

- upper back discomfort between the shoulder blades
- palpitations
- a feeling of fullness in the neck
- nausea
- abdominal discomfort
- dizziness
- unexplained fatigue
- exhaustion or shortness of breath.

Tissue destruction in MI

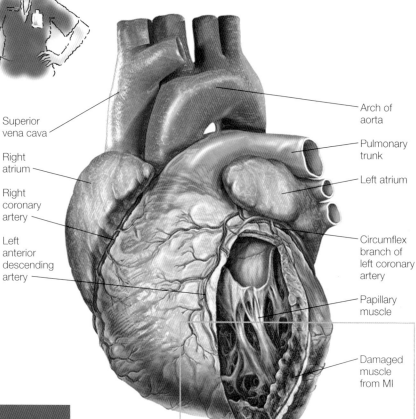

- Arch of aorta
- Pulmonary trunk
- Left atrium
- Circumflex branch of left coronary artery
- Papillary muscle
- Damaged muscle from MI
- Superior vena cava
- Right atrium
- Right coronary artery
- Left anterior descending artery

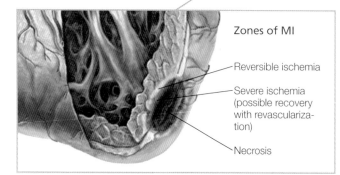

Zones of MI

- Reversible ischemia
- Severe ischemia (possible recovery with revascularization)
- Necrosis

Aortic aneurysm

An aortic aneurysm (AA) is an abnormal dilation in the aortic arterial wall. An aneurysm generally occurs between renal arteries and iliac branches. In a saccular aneurysm, an outpouching occurs in the arterial wall. In fusiform aneurysms, the outpouching appears spindle-shaped and encompasses the entire aortic circumference. In a false aneurysm, the outpouching occurs when the entire vessel wall is injured and leads to a sac formation affecting the artery or heart.

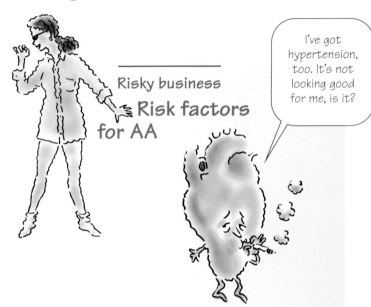

Risky business

Risk factors for AA

I've got hypertension, too. It's not looking good for me, is it?

How it happens

1 Degenerative changes create a focal weakness in the muscular layer of the aorta.

2 The inner and outer layers stretch outward to create a bulge, called an *aneurysm*.

3 Pressure from the blood pulsing through the aorta weakens the vessel wall and enlarges the aneurysm.

Types of aneurysms

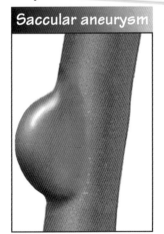

Saccular aneurysm

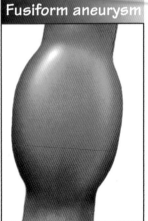

Fusiform aneurysm

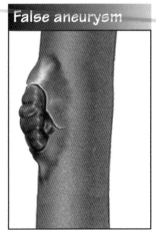

False aneurysm

Dissecting aneurysm

Aneurysms can dissect or rip when bleeding into the weakened artery causes the artery wall to split.

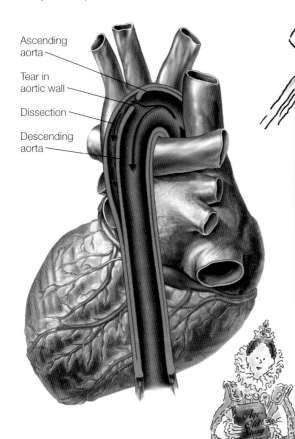

Ascending aorta

Tear in aortic wall

Dissection

Descending aorta

What to look for

Ascending

- Pain
- Bradycardia
- Murmur of aortic insufficiency
- Pericardial friction rub
- Unequal carotid and radial pulses
- Different blood pressures in right and left arms
- Jugular vein distention

Descending

- Pain (suddenly between shoulder blades and chest)
- Hoarseness
- Dyspnea and stridor
- Dysphagia
- Dry cough

Abdominal

- Systolic bruit over aorta
- Tenderness on deep palpation
- Lumbar pain radiating to flank and groin

Age-old story

Age alert for AA

Ascending AAs are usually seen in hypertensive men younger than age 60.

Descending AAs may occur in young patients after a traumatic chest injury or after infection but are most common in elderly men with hypertension.

Cardiac tamponade

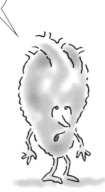
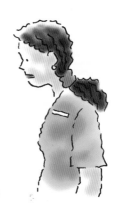

I tell ya, sometimes the pressure is too much.

Cardiac tamponade is a rapid, unchecked increase in pressure in the pericardial sac. This compresses the heart, impairs diastolic filling, and reduces cardiac output.

How it happens

Cardiac tamponade usually results from blood or fluid that accumulates in the pericardial sac and compresses the heart. This compression obstructs blood flow to the ventricles and reduces the amount of blood pumped out of the heart with each contraction. Possible causes include Dressler's syndrome, MI, pericarditis, malignant effusions, or a reaction to certain drugs, such as procainamide (Pronestyl) or hydralazine (Apresoline).

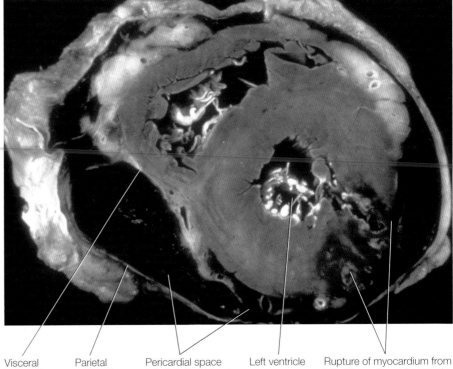

Visceral pericardium

Parietal pericardium

Pericardial space full of clotted blood

Left ventricle

Rupture of myocardium from MI with cardiac cell necrosis

What to look for

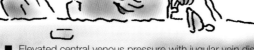

There are three classic signs of cardiac tamponade.

- Elevated central venous pressure with jugular vein distention
- Muffled heart sounds
- Pulsus paradoxus (inspiratory drop in systemic blood pressure greater than 15 mm Hg)

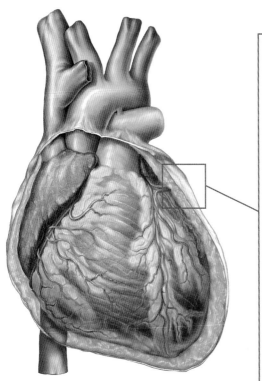

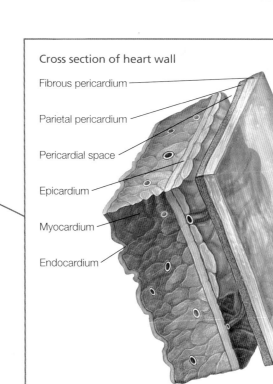

Cross section of heart wall

Fibrous pericardium

Parietal pericardium

Pericardial space

Epicardium

Myocardium

Endocardium

Cardiogenic shock

Cardiogenic shock is a commonly fatal complication of various acute and chronic disorders that impair the heart's ability to maintain adequate tissue perfusion. It can result from any condition that causes significant left ventricular dysfunction and reduced cardiac output, with the most common cause being acute MI.

How it happens

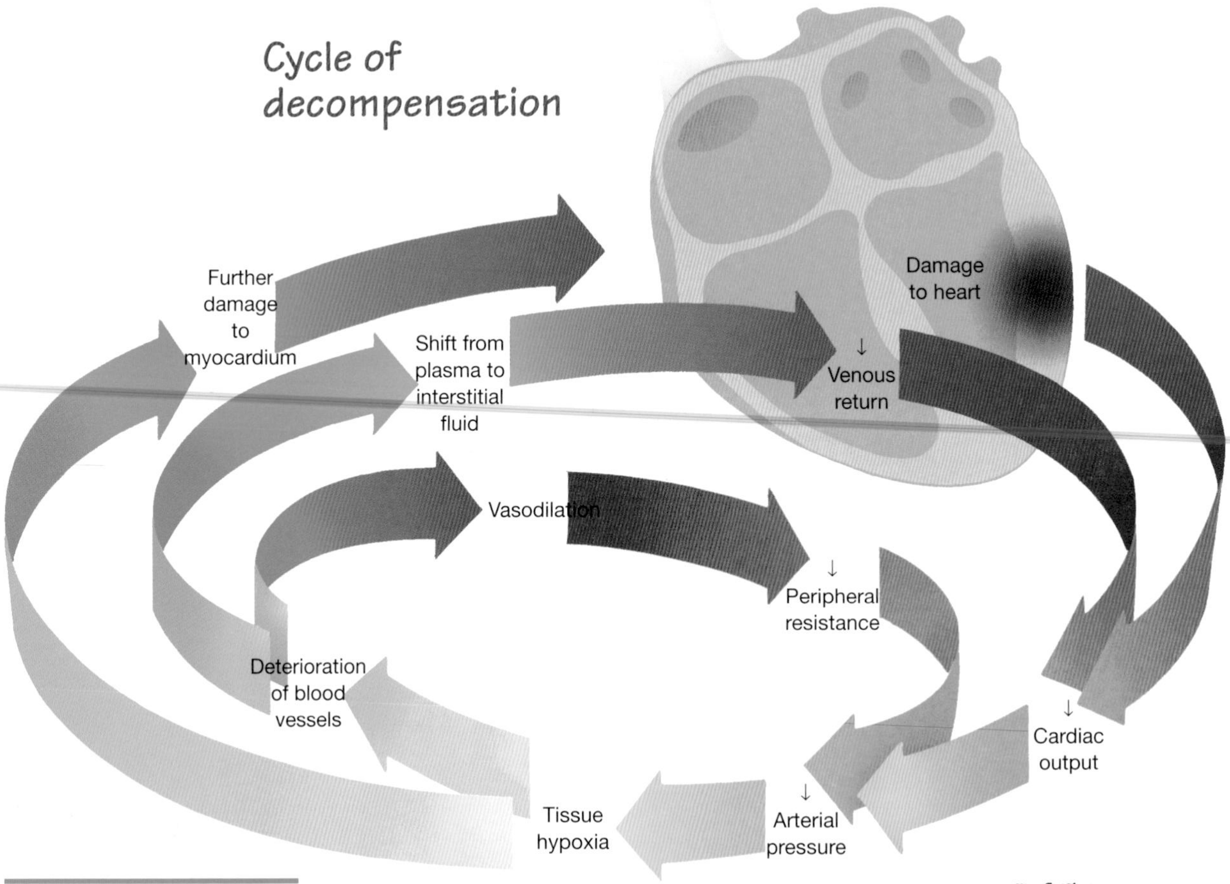

Cycle of decompensation

Further damage to myocardium

Shift from plasma to interstitial fluid

Damage to heart

↓ Venous return

Vasodilation

↓ Peripheral resistance

Deterioration of blood vessels

↓ Cardiac output

Tissue hypoxia

↓ Arterial pressure

What to look for

- Cyanosis
- Metabolic acidosis
- Cool, clammy skin
- Weak, thready pulse

INCREASED
- Heart rate
- Respiration
- Pulmonary artery pressure and pulmonary artery wedge pressure

DECREASED
- Systolic pressure (< 80 mm Hg)
- Urine output (< 20 ml/hour)
- Cardiac index
- Pulse pressure
- Oxygen saturation

Cardiomyopathy
Dilated

Dilated cardiomyopathy is a disease of heart muscle fibers. It usually isn't diagnosed until it has reached an advanced stage and the prognosis is generally poor.

How it happens

Dilated cardiomyopathy results from damage to cardiac muscle fibers. The resulting loss of muscle tone grossly dilates all four chambers of the heart, giving the heart a globular shape.

What to look for

- Shortness of breath
- Orthopnea
- Dyspnea on exertion
- Fatigue
- Dry cough at night
- Peripheral edema
- Hepatomegaly
- Jugular vein distention
- Weight gain
- Peripheral cyanosis
- Tachycardia
- Pansystolic murmur
- S_3 and S_4 gallop rhythms
- Irregular pulse
- Decreased renal function

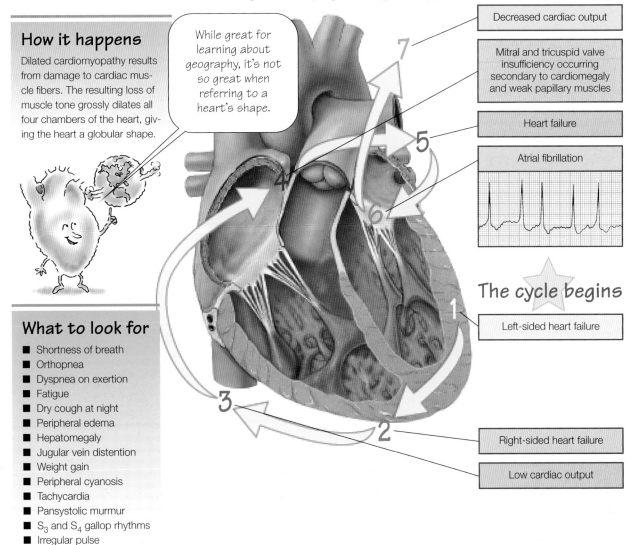

While great for learning about geography, it's not so great when referring to a heart's shape.

Decreased cardiac output

7

Mitral and tricuspid valve insufficiency occurring secondary to cardiomegaly and weak papillary muscles

5

Heart failure

Atrial fibrillation

6

The cycle begins

1

Left-sided heart failure

4

3

2

Right-sided heart failure

Low cardiac output

Cardiomyopathy
Hypertrophic

Hypertrophic cardiomyopathy is a primary disease of cardiac muscle and the interventricular septum of the heart that mainly affects diastolic function.

How it happens

About 50% of the time, hypertrophic cardiomyopathy is transmitted as an autosomal dominant trait. Other causes aren't known.

The damage is done

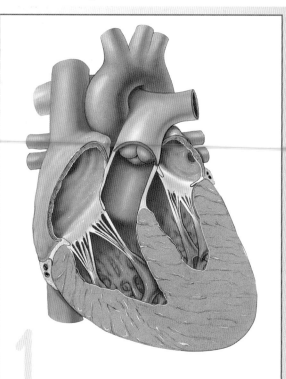

1

The left ventricle and interventricular septum hypertrophy and become stiff, noncompliant, and unable to relax during ventricular filling.

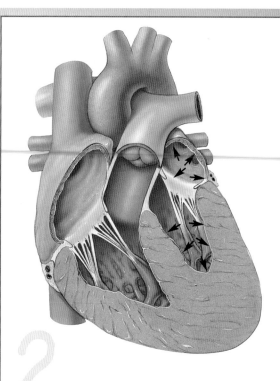

2

As the ventricle's ability to fill decreases, the pressure increases and left atrial and pulmonary venous pressures rise.

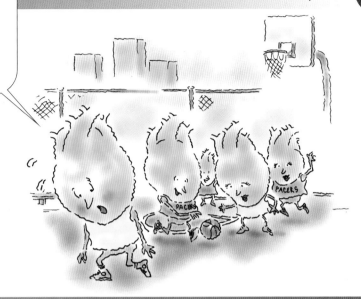

Fifty percent of all sudden deaths in competitive athletes are caused by hypertrophic obstructive cardiomyopathy. Good enough reason for me to take a break!

What to look for

■ Systolic ejection murmur along the left sternal border and at the apex
■ Angina
■ Syncope
■ Activity intolerance
■ Abrupt arterial pulse
■ Irregular pulse (atrial fibrillation)

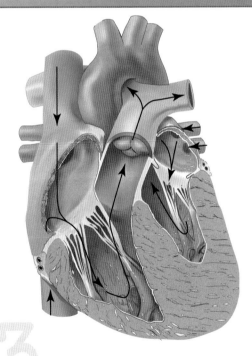

3

The left ventricle forcefully contracts but can't sufficiently relax.

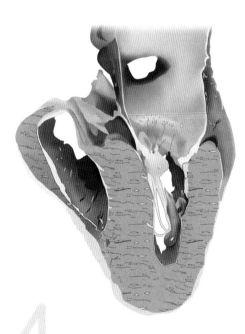

4

The anterior leaflet of the mitral valve is drawn toward the interventricular septum as the blood is forcefully ejected. Early closure of the outflow tract results because of the decreasing ejection fraction.

Cardiomyopathy
Restrictive

Restrictive cardiomyopathy is a disease of heart muscle fibers.
It's irreversible and severe.

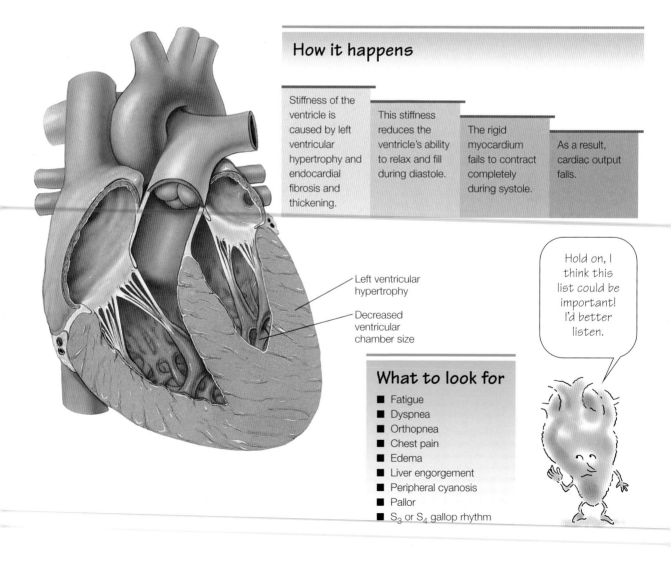

How it happens

Stiffness of the ventricle is caused by left ventricular hypertrophy and endocardial fibrosis and thickening.

This stiffness reduces the ventricle's ability to relax and fill during diastole.

The rigid myocardium fails to contract completely during systole.

As a result, cardiac output falls.

Left ventricular hypertrophy

Decreased ventricular chamber size

Hold on, I think this list could be important! I'd better listen.

What to look for

- Fatigue
- Dyspnea
- Orthopnea
- Chest pain
- Edema
- Liver engorgement
- Peripheral cyanosis
- Pallor
- S_3 or S_4 gallop rhythm

Coronary artery disease

If excessive amounts of fat circulate in the blood, fatty deposits (called *plaques*) can accumulate in the arteries. This buildup, called *atherosclerosis*, causes the vessels to narrow or become obstructed.

How it happens

Coronary artery disease (CAD) results when atherosclerotic plaque fills the lumens of the coronary arteries and obstructs blood flow to the heart, diminishing the supply of oxygen and nutrients to the heart tissue.

What to look for

- Angina
- Nausea and vomiting
- Cool extremities
- Diaphoresis
- Pallor

Coronary arteries

Coronary arteries supply blood to heart tissue. They originate from the aorta.

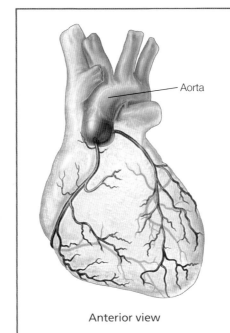

Aorta

Anterior view

Normal coronary artery

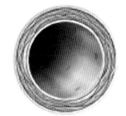

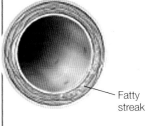

Fatty streak

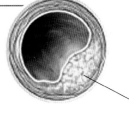

Fibrous plaque

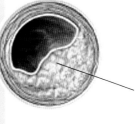

Complicated plaque

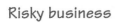

Risky business
Risk factors for CAD

Rising low-density lipoprotein (LDL) and triglyceride levels—LDLs should be less than 130 mg/dl, triglycerides less than 200 mg/dl.

Inadequate control of hypertension, diabetes, and obesity; diet, exercise, and lifestyle changes are key to regaining control.

Sex—CAD is more common in men until after age 75.

Kinfolk—Heredity is a nonmodifiable risk factor.

Smoking—The sooner stopped, the better.

Endocarditis

Endocarditis (also known as *infective* or *bacterial endocarditis*) is an infection of the endocardium, heart valves, or cardiac prosthesis resulting from bacterial or fungal invasion.

How it happens

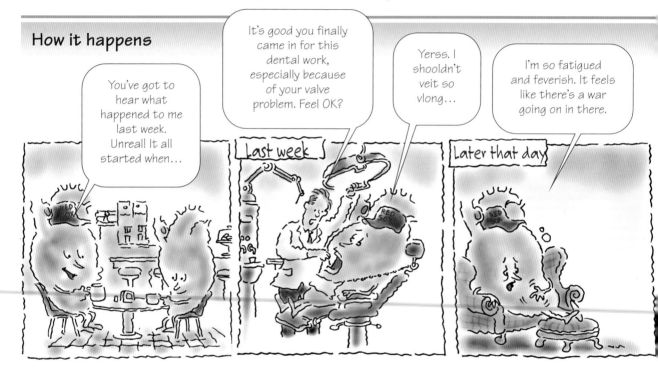

What to look for

- Malaise
- Weakness
- Fatigue
- Weight loss
- Anorexia
- Arthralgia
- Night sweats
- Chills
- Valvular insufficiency
- Intermittent fever that may recur for weeks (in 90% of patients)

Bacterial endocarditis

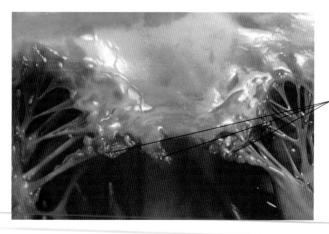

Vegetation destroying valve leaflets

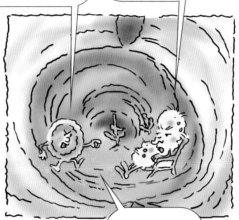

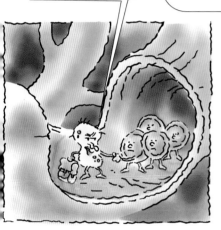

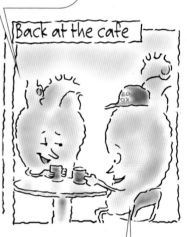

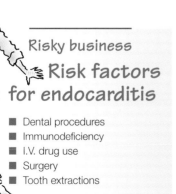

Heart failure

Heart failure is a syndrome that occurs when the heart can't pump enough blood to meet the body's metabolic needs, resulting in intravascular and interstitial volume overload and poor tissue perfusion. Heart failure may be classified as right-sided or left-sided.

5 The right ventricle may now become stressed because it's pumping against greater pulmonary vascular resistance and left ventricular pressure.
- You may note worsening symptoms.

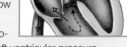

4 Because the left ventricle can't handle the increased venous return, fluid pools in the pulmonary circulation, worsening pulmonary edema.
- You may note decreased breath sounds, dullness on percussion, crackles, and orthopnea.

How it happens

To the left!

3 Rising capillary pressure pushes sodium (Na) and water (H_2O) into the interstitial space, causing pulmonary edema.
- You may note coughing, subclavian retractions, crackles, tachypnea, elevated pulmonary artery pressure, diminished pulmonary compliance, and increased partial pressure of carbon dioxide.

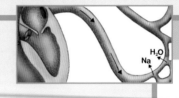

H_2O
Na

Grab your sidewalk chalk and let's hop around these two pages to learn about heart failure!

2 Blood pools in the ventricle and atrium and eventually backs up into the pulmonary veins and capillaries.
- You may note dyspnea on exertion, confusion, dizziness, orthostatic hypotension, decreased peripheral pulses and pulse pressure, cyanosis, and an S_3 gallop.

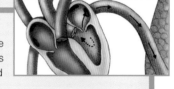

1 Increased workload and end-diastolic volume enlarge the left ventricle.
- You may note increased heart rate, pale and cool skin, tingling in the extremities, decreased cardiac output, and arrhythmias.

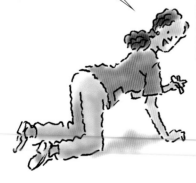

Start

6 The stressed right ventricle enlarges with the formation of stretched tissue.
■ You may note increased heart rate, cool skin, cyanosis, decreased cardiac output, dyspnea, and palpitations.

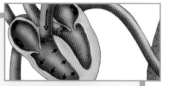

7 Blood pools in the right ventricle and right atrium. The backed up blood causes pressure and congestion in the vena cava and systemic circulation.
■ You may note increased central venous pressure, jugular vein distention, and hepatojugular reflux.

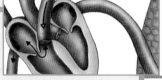

To the right!

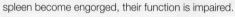

8 Backed up blood distends the visceral veins, especially the hepatic vein. As the liver and spleen become engorged, their function is impaired.
■ You may note anorexia, nausea, abdominal pain, palpable liver and spleen, weakness, and dyspnea secondary to abdominal distention.

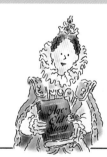

9 Rising capillary pressure forces excess fluid from the capillaries into the interstitial space.
■ You may note edema, weight gain, and nocturia.

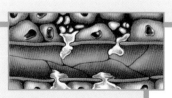

Finish

Age-old story

Heart failure in children

In children, heart failure occurs mainly as a result of congenital heart defects. Therefore, treatment guidelines are directed toward the specific cause.

Hyperlipidemia

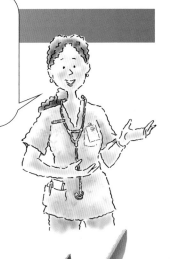

Lipoproteins act as "fat shuttles," transporting cholesterol through the bloodstream.

Hyperlipidemia, also called *hyperproteinemia* or *lipid disorder*, can be primary or secondary and occurs when excess levels of cholesterol, triglycerides, and lipoproteins are present in the blood.

How it happens

Primary
- Inherited autosomal recessive or dominant trait

Secondary
- Diabetes mellitus
- Pancreatitis
- Hypothyroidism
- Renal disease
- Dietary fat intake greater than 40% of total calories; saturated fat intake greater than 10% of total calories; cholesterol intake greater than 300 mg/day
- Habitual excessive alcohol use
- Obesity

What to look for
- Angina
- Nausea and vomiting
- Cool extremities
- Diaphoresis
- Pallor
- Xanthomas

A closer look

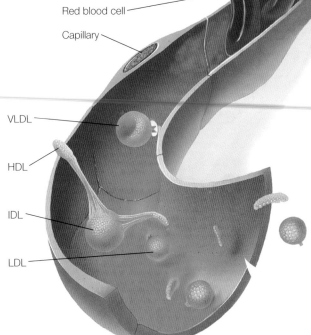

Cholesterol transport in the blood

Very-low-density lipoprotein (VLDL) travels through the bloodstream, attaching to the lining of the capillaries. There, its fatty core of cholesterol is drawn out.

Red blood cell

Capillary

How cholesterol is made

The smaller particles of intermediate-density lipoprotein (IDL) that remain in the blood shed tiny disklike particles of high-density lipoprotein (HDL; good cholesterol).

VLDL

HDL

IDL

LDL

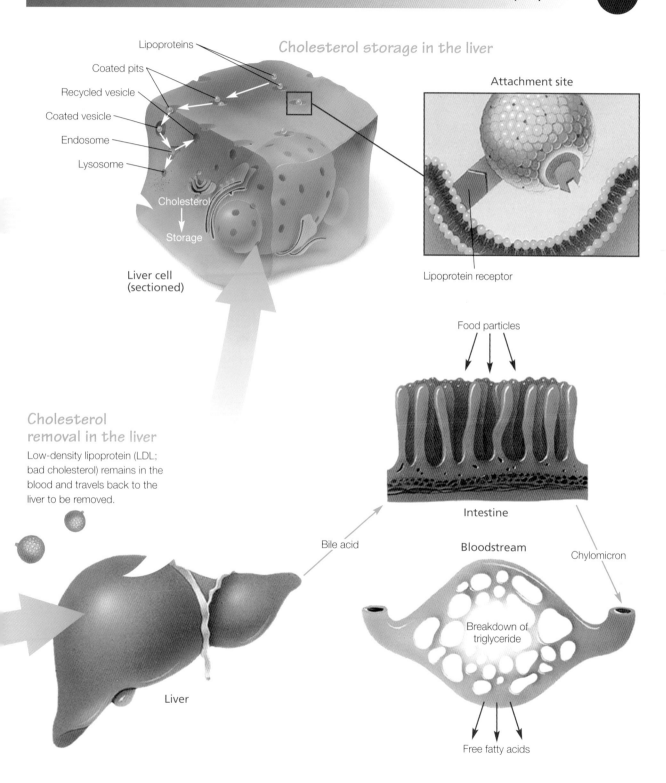

Cholesterol storage in the liver

Lipoproteins
Coated pits
Recycled vesicle
Coated vesicle
Endosome
Lysosome
Cholesterol
Storage
Liver cell
(sectioned)

Attachment site

Lipoprotein receptor

Cholesterol removal in the liver

Low-density lipoprotein (LDL; bad cholesterol) remains in the blood and travels back to the liver to be removed.

Bile acid

Liver

Food particles

Intestine

Bloodstream

Chylomicron

Breakdown of triglyceride

Free fatty acids

Hypertension

Hypertension is intermittent or sustained elevation of systolic blood pressure greater than 139 mm Hg or diastolic blood pressure greater than 89 mm Hg. Hypertension occurs as essential (primary) hypertension or as secondary hypertension.

Risky business

Risk factors for primary hypertension

- Diabetes mellitus
- Family history
- Advancing age
- Obesity
- Sedentary lifestyle
- Stress
- Smoking
- High intake of sodium, saturated fats, and alcohol

How it happens

Several theories exist.

1 Changes in the arteriolar bed cause increased total peripheral resistance (TPR).

2 Abnormally increased tone in the sympathetic nervous system causes increased TPR.

3 Increased arteriolar thickening caused by genetic factors leads to TPR.

4 Abnormal renin release results in formation of angiotensin II, which constricts the arterioles and increases blood volume.

What to look for

- Elevated blood pressure
- Bruits over abdominal aorta or carotid, renal, and femoral arteries
- Dizziness
- Confusion
- Fatigue
- Blurred vision
- Nocturia
- Edema

Angiotensin II

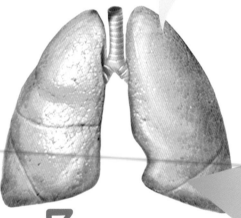

3 Angiotensin I is converted to angiotensin II (a potent vasoconstrictor) in lungs.

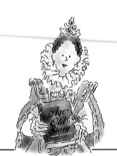

Age-old story

Age and systolic hypertension

Elderly people may have isolated systolic hypertension, in which just the systolic blood pressure is elevated, because atherosclerosis causes a loss of elasticity in large arteries.

As you get older, you lose elasticity—in your face and in your arteries!

Understanding hypertension

Aldosterone

5 Aldosterone causes sodium and water retention.

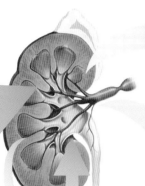

1 Kidneys release renin into the bloodstream.

Renin

6 Retained sodium and water increase blood volume.

Aldosterone

4 Angiotensin II causes arteriolar constriction and aldosterone secretion.

2 Renin helps convert angiotensin to angiotensin I in liver.

Angiotensin

Angiotensin I

8 Increased blood volume and vascular resistance cause hypertension.

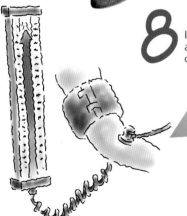

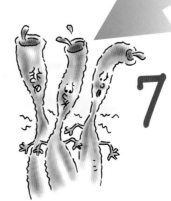

7 Arteriolar constriction increases peripheral vascular resistance.

Hypovolemic shock

In hypovolemic shock, reduced intravascular volume causes circulatory dysfunction and inadequate tissue perfusion. It's commonly caused by acute blood loss—about 20% of total volume—that can result from:

■ GI bleeding, internal or external hemorrhage, or a condition that reduces circulating intravascular volume or levels of other fluids
■ intestinal obstruction
■ peritonitis
■ acute pancreatitis
■ dehydration from excessive perspiration, severe diarrhea, protracted vomiting, diabetes insipidus, diuresis, or inadequate fluid intake.

Third-space fluid shift, which can occur in the abdominal cavity (ascites), pleural cavity, or pericardial sac, can also cause hypovolemic shock.

How it happens

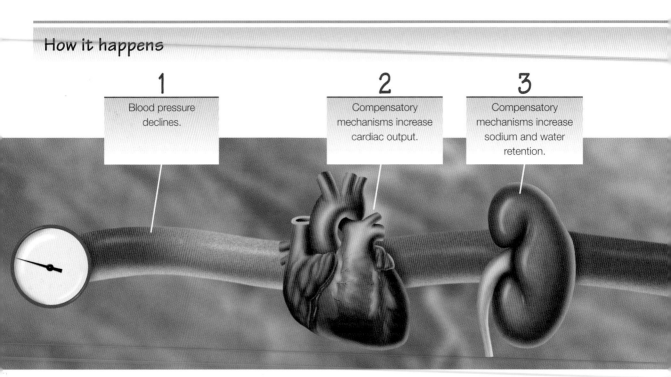

1 Blood pressure declines.

2 Compensatory mechanisms increase cardiac output.

3 Compensatory mechanisms increase sodium and water retention.

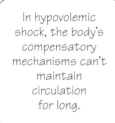

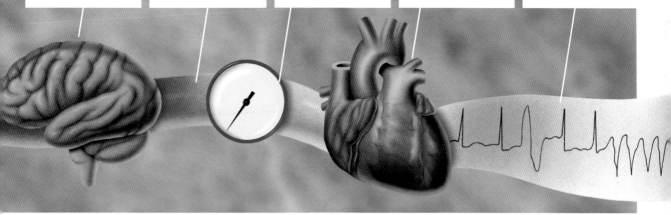

4
Compensatory mechanisms (release of antidiuretic hormone) stimulate thirst.

5
Compensatory mechanisms fail.

6
Blood pressure falls, and tissue perfusion is impaired.

7
Oxygen and nutrient delivery to cells decreases.

8
Cardiac ischemia and arrhythmias may develop.

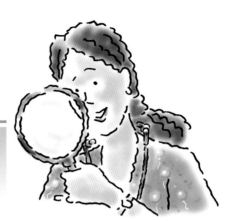

What to look for

- Cyanosis
- Metabolic acidosis
- Cool, clammy skin
- Weak, thready pulse

INCREASED

- Heart rate
- Respiration
- Urine specific gravity
- Potassium, creatinine, and blood urea nitrogen levels

DECREASED

- Sensorium
- Pulse pressure
- Urine output (less than 25 ml/hour)
- Blood pressure
- Central venous pressure, pulmonary artery pressure, and pulmonary artery wedge pressure
- Hemoglobin level
- Hematocrit

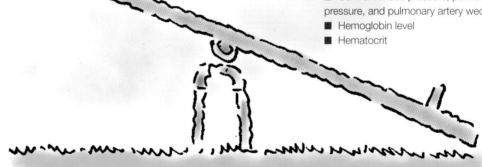

Myocarditis

Myocarditis is focal or diffuse inflammation of the cardiac muscle (myocardium). It may be acute or chronic and can occur at any age.

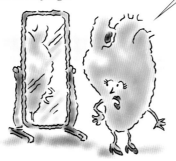

Honestly, does this look flabby to you?

How it happens

Damage to the myocardium occurs when an infectious organism triggers an autoimmune, cellular, and humoral reaction. The resulting inflammation may lead to hypertrophy, fibrosis, and inflammatory changes of the myocardium and conduction system. The heart muscle weakens and contractility is reduced. The heart muscle becomes flabby and dilated and pinpoint hemorrhages may develop.

Normal heart anatomy

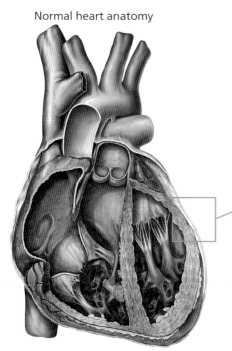

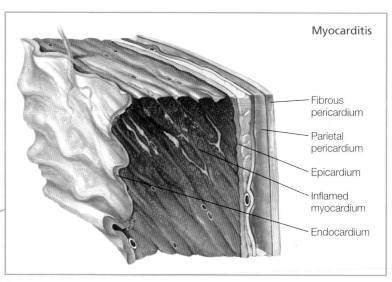

Myocarditis

- Fibrous pericardium
- Parietal pericardium
- Epicardium
- Inflamed myocardium
- Endocardium

What to look for

- Fatigue
- Dyspnea
- Palpitations
- Fever
- Mild, continuous pressure or soreness in the chest
- Tachycardia
- S_3 and S_4 gallops
- Murmur of mitral insufficiency may be heard, if papillary muscles are involved

Pericarditis

Pericarditis is an inflammation of the pericardium. Acute pericarditis can be fibrinous or effusive, with purulent, serous, or hemorrhagic exudate. Chronic constrictive pericarditis is characterized by dense fibrous pericardial thickening.

How it happens

- Bacterial, fungal, or viral infection
- Neoplasms
- High-dose radiation to the chest
- Autoimmune disease such as systemic lupus erythematosus
- Drugs, such as hydralazine or procainamide
- Infection after cardiac surgery

The inflammatory process in pericarditis

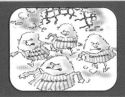 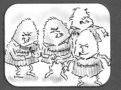 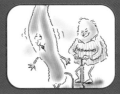 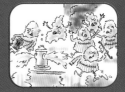 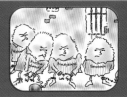

1 Pericardial tissue damaged by bacteria or other substances releases chemical mediators of inflammation into the surrounding tissue.

2 Friction occurs as the inflamed pericardial layers rub against each other.

3 Histamines and other chemical mediators dilate vessels and increase vessel permeability.

4 Fluids and protein (including fibrinogen) leak into the tissues, causing extracellular edema. Macrophages, neutrophils, and monocytes in the tissue begin to phagocytose the invading bacteria.

5 Gradually, the space fills with an exudate composed of necrotic tissue, dead and dying bacteria, neutrophils, and macrophages. These products are eventually reabsorbed into healthy tissue.

What to look for

- Pericardial friction rub
- Sharp, sudden pain starting at the sternum and radiating to the neck, shoulders, and arms
- Shallow, rapid respirations
- Mild fever
- Dyspnea
- Orthopnea
- Tachycardia
- Muffled and distant heart sounds
- Fluid retention
- Ascites
- Hepatomegaly
- Jugular vein distention

> Common symptoms of pericarditis are pain at the sternum and shallow, rapid respirations.

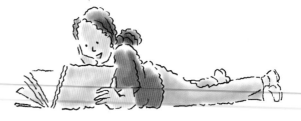

Valvular heart disease
Aortic insufficiency

> Jiminy Cricket! I think someone forgot to shut off the aortic valve!

Aortic insufficiency is the incomplete closure of the aortic valve. It can be acute or chronic and is usually caused by scarring or retraction of valve leaflets.

In aortic insufficiency, blood flows back into the left ventricle during diastole, causing fluid overload in the ventricle, which dilates and hypertrophies. The excess volume causes fluid overload in the left atrium and, finally, in the pulmonary system. Left-sided heart failure and pulmonary edema eventually result.

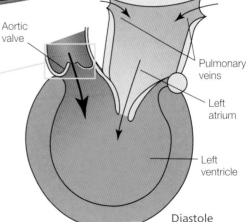

How it happens

Acute

- Endocarditis
- Chest trauma
- Prosthetic valve malfunction
- Acute ascending aortic dissection

Chronic

- Hypertension
- Rheumatic fever
- Marfan syndrome
- Ankylosing spondylitis
- Syphilis
- Ventricular septal defect

What to look for

- Pulmonary congestion
- Shock
- Dyspnea
- Orthopnea
- Paroxysmal nocturnal dyspnea
- Fatigue
- Exercise intolerance
- Pulsating nail beds
- S_3 heart sound
- Angina
- Palpitations
- Widened pulse pressure
- Diastolic blowing murmur at left sternal border

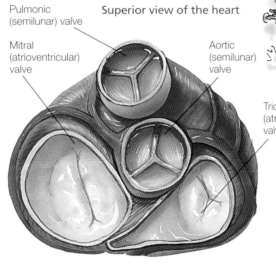

Superior view of the heart

Pulmonic (semilunar) valve

Mitral (atrioventricular) valve

Aortic (semilunar) valve

Tricuspid (atrioventricular) valve

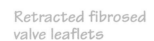

Retracted fibrosed valve leaflets

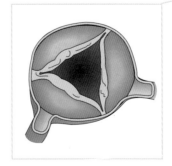

Aortic insufficiency

Aortic valve

Pulmonary veins

Left atrium

Left ventricle

Diastole

Valvular heart disease

Aortic stenosis

Aortic stenosis is a narrowing of the aortic valve. It may be classified as:

Acquired

Rheumatic.

Increased left ventricular pressure tries to overcome the resistance of the narrowed valvular opening. The added workload increases the demand for oxygen, and diminished cardiac output causes poor coronary artery perfusion, ischemia of the left ventricle, and left-sided heart failure.

How it happens

Aortic stenosis can occur as a result of:
- idiopathic fibrosis and calcification
- congenital aortic bicuspid valve
- rheumatic fever
- atherosclerosis.

What to look for

Angina

Syncope

Dyspnea

Aortic valve stenosis

Aortic valve

Thickened and stenotic valve leaflets

Pulmonary veins

Left atrium

Mitral valve

Left ventricle

Systole

Valvular heart disease
Mitral insufficiency

> There's too much flowing from the left ventricle into the left atrium. I can't accommodate all of this backflow!

An abnormality of the mitral leaflets, mitral annulus, chordae tendineae, papillary muscles, left atrium, or left ventricle can lead to mitral insufficiency.

Blood from the left ventricle flows back into the left atrium during systole, causing the atrium to enlarge to accommodate the backflow. As a result, the left ventricle also dilates to accommodate the increased blood volume from the atrium and to compensate for diminishing cardiac output. Ventricular hypertrophy and increased end-diastolic pressure result in increased pulmonary artery pressure, eventually leading to left-sided and right-sided heart failure.

How it happens

Mitral insufficiency can occur as a result of:
- rheumatic fever
- mitral valve prolapse
- hypertrophic obstructive cardiomyopathy
- myocardial infarction
- ruptured chordae tendineae
- transposition of great arteries.

What to look for

- Exertional dyspnea
- Paroxysmal nocturnal dyspnea
- Orthopnea
- Weakness
- Fatigue
- Palpitations
- Peripheral edema
- Jugular vein distention
- Ascites
- Hepatomegaly (right-sided heart failure)
- Crackles
- Atrial fibrillation
- A loud S_1 or opening snap and a diastolic murmur at the apex

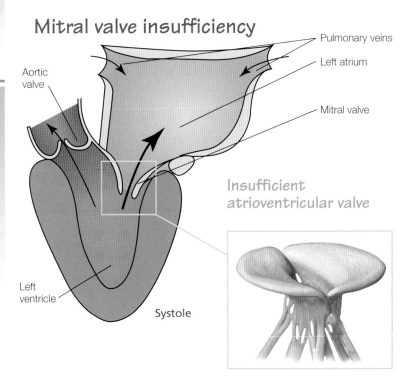

Mitral valve insufficiency

Pulmonary veins

Left atrium

Mitral valve

Aortic valve

Left ventricle

Systole

Insufficient atrioventricular valve

Valvular heart disease

Mitral prolapse

Mitral valve prolapse is a billowing and subsequent improper closing of the mitral valve. It occurs more frequently in women than in men.

How it happens

Mitral valve prolapse can occur as a result of:
- autosomal dominant inheritance
- genetic or environmental interruption of valve development during week 5 or 6 of gestation
- inherited connective tissue disorders, such as Ehlers-Danlos syndrome, Marfan syndrome, and osteogenesis imperfecta.

What to look for

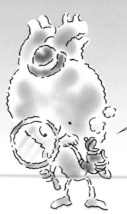

Dizziness, syncope, palpitations, chest pain, and heart murmur? Just as I suspected— mitral prolapse, I presume.

memory board

In valvular heart disease, the heart's aortic and mitral valves can be subjected to three types of disruption. To help you remember them, just think **SIP**:

Stenosis

Insufficiency

Prolapse.

Cross section of left ventricle

Mitral valve prolapse

A view of the mitral valve from the left atrium shows redundant and deformed leaflets that billow into the left atrial cavity.

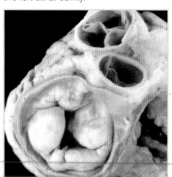

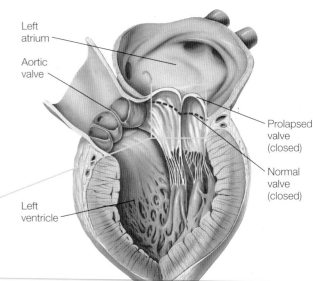

Left atrium

Aortic valve

Left ventricle

Prolapsed valve (closed)

Normal valve (closed)

Valvular heart disease
Mitral stenosis

How it happens

Mitral stenosis can occur as a result of:
- rheumatic fever
- congenital abnormalities
- atrial myxoma
- endocarditis
- adverse effect of fenfluramine and phentermine diet drug combination. (This drug combination has been removed from the U.S. drug market.)

Mitral valve stenosis

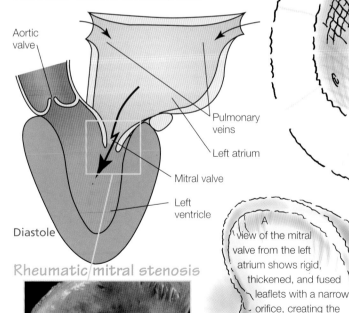

Aortic valve

Pulmonary veins

Left atrium

Mitral valve

Left ventricle

Diastole

Rheumatic mitral stenosis

> Well, I'd say that's an inadequate filling. You won't get too much output from me!

Mitral stenosis involves narrowing of the valve by valvular abnormalities, fibrosis, or calcification that obstructs blood flow from the left atrium to the left ventricle. Consequently, left atrial volume and pressure rise and the chamber dilates. Greater resistance to blood flow causes pulmonary hypertension, right ventricular hypertrophy, and right-sided heart failure. Also, inadequate filling of the left ventricle produces low cardiac output.

A view of the mitral valve from the left atrium shows rigid, thickened, and fused leaflets with a narrow orifice, creating the characteristic "fish mouth" appearance of rheumatic mitral stenosis.

What to look for

- Orthopnea
- Dyspnea
- Fatigue
- Angina
- Palpitations
- Peripheral edema
- Jugular vein distention
- Hepatomegaly
(right-sided heart failure)
- Tachycardia
- Crackles
- Pulmonary edema
- Holosystolic murmur at the apex, a possible split S_2, and an S_3

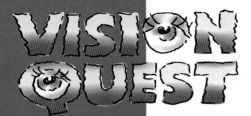
VISION QUEST

Matchmaker

Match the definitions given here with their corresponding disorders.

1. Inflammation of the pericardium ____
2. An infection of the endocardium, heart valves, or cardiac prosthesis ____
3. An abnormal dilation in the aortic arterial wall ____
4. An unchecked increase in pressure in the pericardial sac ____
5. Narrowing of the aortic valve ____
6. A disease of heart muscle fibers ____

A. Cardiomyopathy
B. Aortic stenosis
C. Cardiac tamponade
D. Endocarditis
E. Aortic aneurysm
F. Pericarditis

Rebus riddle

Solve the riddle to find an important fact about coronary artery disease.

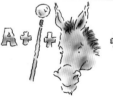 + EE + S That A + + 8

IN THE + ER + EEE R + ED .

3 Respiratory disorders

> You gotta bring your lungs for this chapter. Aaaaa-ayyyahhhh!

Acute respiratory distress syndrome

Acute respiratory distress syndrome (ARDS) is a form of pulmonary edema that can quickly lead to acute respiratory failure. Also known as *shock* or *stiff, white, wet,* or *Da Nang lung*, ARDS may follow a direct or indirect lung injury. It's difficult to diagnose and can prove fatal within 48 hours of onset if not promptly diagnosed and treated. (Ventricular fibrillation or standstill may occur.) Mortality associated with ARDS remains at 50% to 70%.

How it happens

Shock, sepsis, and trauma are the most common causes of ARDS. Trauma-related factors, such as fat emboli, pulmonary contusions, and multiple transfusions, may increase the likelihood that microemboli will develop.

A closer look

Phase 1

In *phase 1,* injury reduces normal blood flow to the lungs. Platelets aggregate and release histamine (H), serotonin (S), and bradykinin (B).

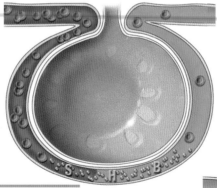

Phase 2

In *phase 2,* those substances—especially histamine—inflame and damage the alveolocapillary membrane, increasing capillary permeability. Fluids then shift into the interstitial space.

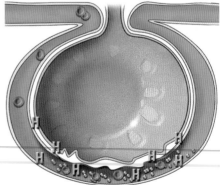

Phase 3

In *phase 3,* as capillary permeability increases, proteins and fluids leak out, increasing interstitial osmotic pressure and causing pulmonary edema.

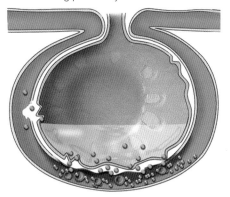

Phase 4

In *phase 4,* decreased blood flow and fluids in the alveoli damage surfactant and impair the cell's ability to produce more. As a result, alveoli collapse, impeding gas exchange and decreasing lung compliance.

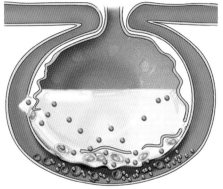

Phase 5

In *phase 5,* sufficient oxygen can't cross the alveolocapillary membrane, but carbon dioxide (CO_2) can and is lost with every exhalation. Oxygen (O_2) and CO_2 levels decrease in the blood.

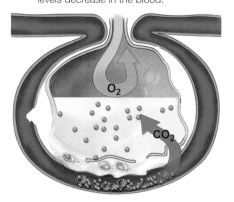

Phase 6

In *phase 6,* pulmonary edema worsens, inflammation leads to fibrosis, and gas exchange is further impeded.

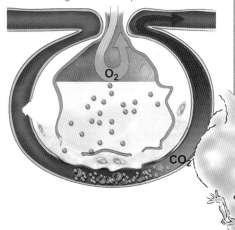

What to look for

- Rapid, shallow breathing
- Dyspnea
- Hypoxemia
- Intercostal and supra-sternal retractions
- Crackles
- Rhonchi
- Restlessness
- Apprehension
- Mental sluggishness
- Motor dysfunction
- Tachycardia

Severe ARDS

- Hypotension
- Decreased urine output
- Respiratory and metabolic acidosis

memory board

Antibiotics

Respiratory support

Diuretics

Situate the patient in the prone position.

Use the abbreviation for ARDS to remember key treatments.

Asthma

Asthma is a chronic reactive airway disorder that can present as an acute attack. It causes episodic airway obstruction resulting from bronchospasms, increased mucus secretion, and mucosal edema. Asthma is one type of chronic obstructive pulmonary disease (COPD), a long-term pulmonary disease characterized by airflow resistance.

Cases of asthma continue to rise. It currently affects an estimated 17 million Americans; children account for 4.8 million asthma sufferers in the United States.

A case of exposure

1st exposure

1 Allergens may enter through the nose and mouth.

Ragweed

Pollen grains (allergens)

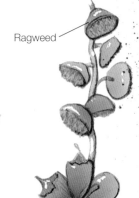

Ragweed

Age-old story

Age and asthma

Although asthma strikes at any age, about 50% of patients are younger than age 10; twice as many boys as girls are affected in this age-group. One-third of patients develop asthma from ages 10 to 30, and the incidence is the same in both sexes in this age-group.

How it happens

2 Allergens are absorbed into the tissues.

Allergens

Immune cell

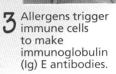

3 Allergens trigger immune cells to make immunoglobulin (Ig) E antibodies.

IgE antibody

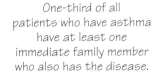
One-third of all patients who have asthma have at least one immediate family member who also has the disease.

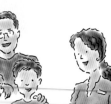

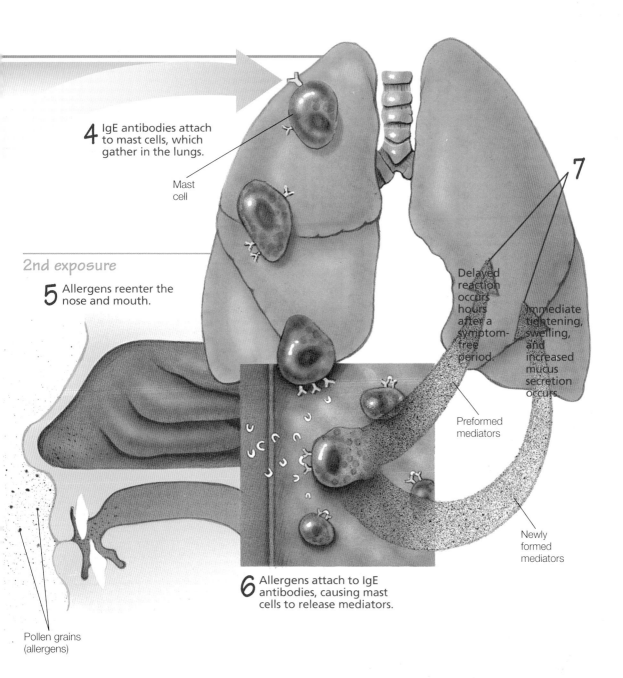

4 IgE antibodies attach to mast cells, which gather in the lungs.

Mast cell

2nd exposure

5 Allergens reenter the nose and mouth.

7

Delayed reaction occurs hours after a symptom-free period.

Immediate tightening, swelling, and increased mucus secretion occurs

Preformed mediators

Newly formed mediators

6 Allergens attach to IgE antibodies, causing mast cells to release mediators.

Pollen grains (allergens)

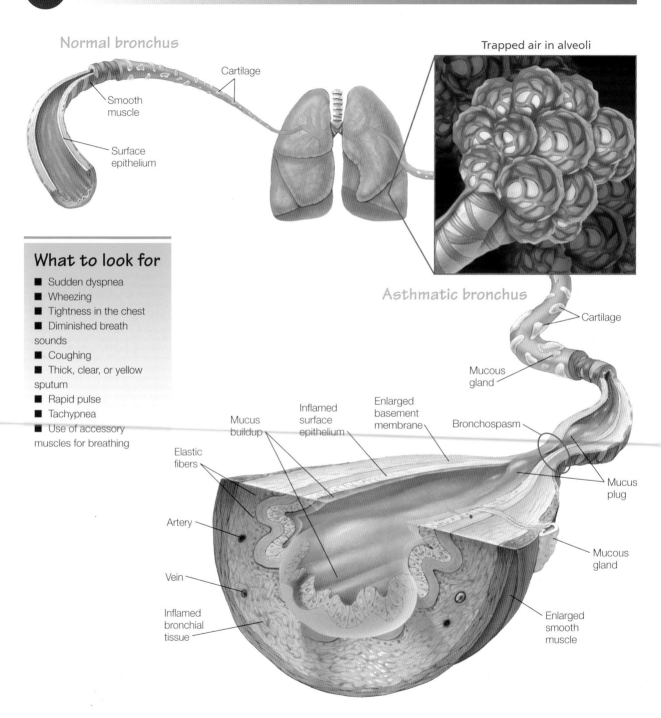

Normal bronchus

Cartilage

Smooth muscle

Surface epithelium

Trapped air in alveoli

Asthmatic bronchus

What to look for

- Sudden dyspnea
- Wheezing
- Tightness in the chest
- Diminished breath sounds
- Coughing
- Thick, clear, or yellow sputum
- Rapid pulse
- Tachypnea
- Use of accessory muscles for breathing

Elastic fibers

Mucus buildup

Inflamed surface epithelium

Enlarged basement membrane

Bronchospasm

Cartilage

Mucous gland

Mucus plug

Artery

Vein

Inflamed bronchial tissue

Mucous gland

Enlarged smooth muscle

Chronic bronchitis

Chronic bronchitis, a form of COPD, is inflammation of the bronchi caused by irritants or infection.

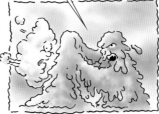

My job as airflow is vital to breathing!

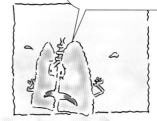

This is my second straight year of hanging around longer than 3 months. I love being a menace!

That mucus is blocking my airflow! Chronic bronchitis can't be far behind!

How it happens

Chronic bronchitis occurs when irritants are inhaled for a prolonged period. The result is resistance in the small airways and severe ventilation-perfusion imbalance that decreases arterial oxygenation.

Patients have a diminished respiratory drive, so they usually hypoventilate. Chronic hypoxia causes the kidneys to produce erythropoietin. This stimulates excessive red blood cell production, leading to polycythemia. The hemoglobin level is high, but the amount of reduced hemoglobin that comes in contact with oxygen is low; therefore, cyanosis is evident.

Healthy bronchi

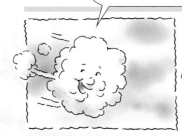

Normal bronchial tube

- Lumen
- Mucus
- Cilia
- Goblet cell
- Mucous glands

Chronic bronchitis

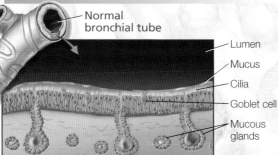

Narrowed bronchial tube

- Lumen
- Excessive mucus retention
- Bacteria
- Damaged cilia
- Increased number of goblet cells
- Enlarged mucous glands

What to look for

- Productive cough
- Dyspnea
- Cyanosis
- Use of accessory muscles for breathing
- Pulmonary hypertension

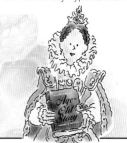

Age-old story

Age and chronic bronchitis

Children of parents who smoke are at higher risk for respiratory tract infection that can lead to chronic bronchitis.

Cor pulmonale

In cor pulmonale, hypertrophy and dilation of the right ventricle develop secondary to a disease affecting the structure or function of the lungs or associated structures.

This condition occurs at the end stage of various chronic disorders of the lungs, pulmonary vessels, chest wall, and respiratory control center.

Cor pulmonale causes about 25% of all types of heart failure. About 85% of patients with cor pulmonale also have COPD, and about 25% of patients with bronchial COPD eventually develop cor pulmonale. It's most common in smokers and middle-age and elderly men; however, incidence in women is rising.

An overview

Although pulmonary restrictive disorders (such as fibrosis or obesity), obstructive disorders (such as bronchitis), or primary vascular disorders (such as recurrent pulmonary emboli) may cause cor pulmonale, these disorders share this common pathway.

How it happens

Cor pulmonale may result from:
- disorders that affect the pulmonary parenchyma
- pulmonary diseases that affect the airways such as COPD
- vascular diseases, such as vasculitis, pulmonary emboli, or external vascular obstruction resulting from a tumor or an aneurysm
- chest wall abnormalities, including such thoracic deformities as kyphoscoliosis and pectus excavatum (funnel chest)
- neuromuscular disorders, such as muscular dystrophy and poliomyelitis
- external factors, such as obesity and living at a high altitude.

Pulmonary disorder

↓

Anatomic alterations in the pulmonary blood vessels and functional alterations in the lung

↓

Increased pulmonary vascular resistance

↓

Pulmonary hypertension

↓

Right ventricular hypertrophy (cor pulmonale)

↓

Heart failure

Cross-section of the heart with cor pulmonale

What to look for

Early
- Chronic, productive cough
- Exertional dyspnea
- Wheezing respirations
- Fatigue and weakness

Progressive
- Dyspnea at rest
- Tachypnea
- Orthopnea
- Dependent edema
- Distended jugular veins
- Hepatomegaly (enlarged, tender liver)
- Hepatojugular reflux (jugular vein distention induced by pressing over the liver)
- Right upper quadrant discomfort
- Tachycardia
- Decreased cardiac output
- Weight gain

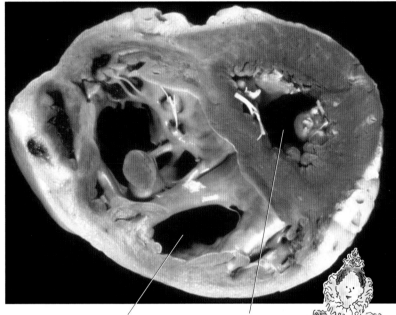

Right ventricle   Left ventricle

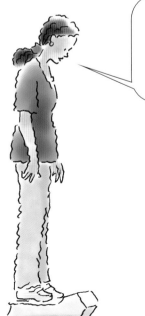

Weight gain is one of the symptoms of progressive cor pulmonale. Best to keep those lungs and heart healthy!

Age-old story

Age and cor pulmonale

In children, cor pulmonale may be a complication of cystic fibrosis, hemosiderosis, upper-airway obstruction, scleroderma, extensive bronchiectasis, neuromuscular diseases that affect respiratory muscles, or abnormalities of the respiratory control area.

Emphysema

A form of COPD, emphysema is the abnormal, permanent enlargement of the acini accompanied by destruction of the alveolar walls. Obstruction results from tissue changes, rather than mucus production, as occurs in asthma and chronic bronchitis.

The distinguishing characteristic of emphysema is airflow limitation caused by a lack of elastic recoil in the lungs.

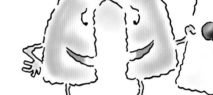

memory board

Asthma

Chronic bronchitis

Emphysema

Need to remember the types of COPD? Remember that you'll need to ACE this one!

How it happens

Emphysema may be caused by a deficiency of alpha$_1$-protease inhibitor or by cigarette smoking.

In emphysema, recurrent inflammation is associated with the release of proteolytic enzymes (enzymes that promote protein splitting by peptide bond hydrolysis) from lung cells. This causes irreversible enlargement of the air spaces distal to the terminal bronchioles. Enlargement of air spaces destroys the alveolar walls, which results in a breakdown of elasticity and the loss of fibrous and muscle tissues, making the lungs less compliant.

Lung changes in emphysema

Alveolus

Smooth muscle

Dilation and destruction of bronchial walls

Loss of lung tissue

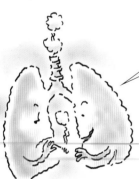

If I keep this up, it's shortness of breath, chronic cough, and wheezing for me!

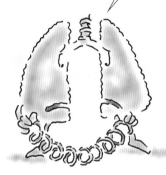

What to look for

- Tachypnea
- Exertional dyspnea
- Barrel-shaped chest
- Prolonged expiration and grunting
- Decreased breath sounds
- Clubbed fingers and toes
- Decreased tactile fremitus
- Decreased chest expansion
- Hyperresonance
- Crackles and wheezing on inspiration

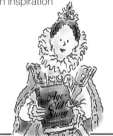

Age-old story

Age and emphysema

Aging is a risk factor for emphysema. Senile emphysema results from degenerative changes; stretching occurs without destruction in the smooth muscle. Connective tissue isn't usually affected.

Air trapping in emphysema

After alveolar walls are damaged or destroyed, they can't support and keep the airways open. The alveolar walls then lose their capability of elastic recoil. Collapse then occurs on expiration, as shown here.

Normal expiration

Note normal recoil and the open bronchiole.

Impaired expiration

Note decreased elastic recoil and a narrowed bronchiole.

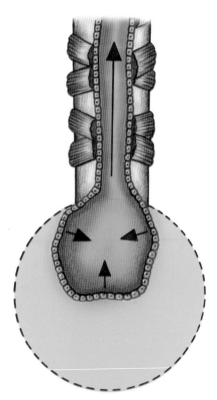

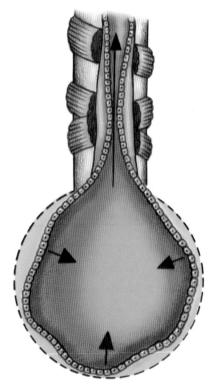

Fat embolism syndrome

Fat embolism syndrome is a rare but potentially fatal problem. It involves pulmonary, cerebral, and cutaneous manifestations and occurs 24 to 48 hours after a traumatic injury.

How it happens

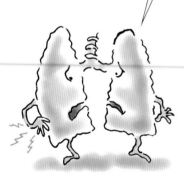

I'd better be on the lookout for fat embolism syndrome in about a day or two...

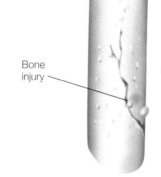

1 Bone marrow from a fractured bone releases fat globules.

Bone injury

What to look for

- Petechiae
- Increased respiratory rate
- Dyspnea
- Accessory muscle use for breathing
- Mental status changes
- Jaundice
- Fever

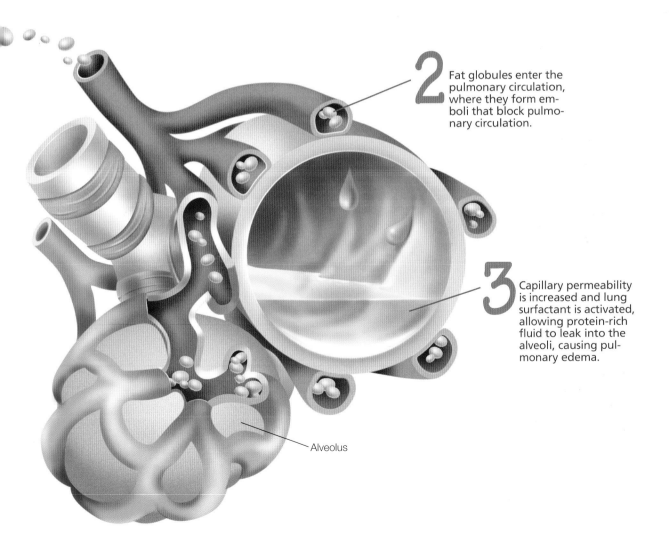

2 Fat globules enter the pulmonary circulation, where they form emboli that block pulmonary circulation.

3 Capillary permeability is increased and lung surfactant is activated, allowing protein-rich fluid to leak into the alveoli, causing pulmonary edema.

Alveolus

Influenza

Influenza, also known as the *flu* or *grippe*, is an acute, highly contagious infection of the respiratory tract. Influenza occurs sporadically or in epidemics (usually during the colder months). Epidemics usually peak in 2 to 3 weeks after initial cases appear and last 2 to 3 months.

> Influenza results from three types of virus.

How it happens

Type A

Type A, the most prevalent, strikes every year, with new serotypes causing epidemics every 3 years.

Type B

Type B also strikes annually but only causes epidemics every 4 to 6 years.

Type C

Type C is endemic and causes only sporadic cases.

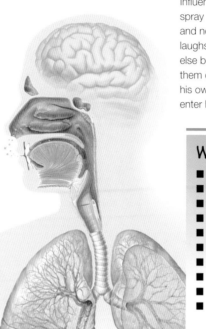

Understanding influenza

Influenza spreads in the droplets that spray out of an infected person's mouth and nose when he sneezes or coughs, laughs, or even talks. When someone else breathes in these droplets or gets them on his hands and then touches his own mouth or nose, the virus can enter his body.

What to look for

- Fever
- Headache
- Fatigue, weakness
- Runny or stuffy nose
- Sneezing
- Sore throat
- Cough
- Chest discomfort
- General aches and pains
- Bronchitis

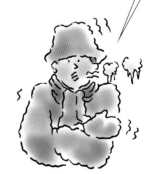

Fever, headache, sneezing…I'm afraid I must have had an unfortunate meeting with some droplets!

Risky business
Risk factors for complications of influenza

- Age 65 and older
- Ages 6 months to 23 months
- Any age with chronic medical conditions
- Pregnancy

Lung cancer

Although lung cancer is largely preventable, it remains the most common cause of cancer death in men and women.

About 80% of lung cancers are non-small-cell lung cancer, which includes three subtypes. The cells in these subtypes differ in size, shape, and chemical makeup and are described here.

Adenocarcinoma	Squamous cell	Large-cell undifferentiated
■ Usually found in the outer region of the lung	■ Commonly linked to a history of smoking ■ Tends to be found centrally, near a bronchus	■ Can appear in any part of the lung ■ Tends to grow and spread quickly

The remaining 20% of lung cancers are small-cell lung cancer. Although the cancer cells in this type of cancer are small, they can multiply quickly and form large tumors that spread to the lymph nodes and other structures, such as the brain, liver, and bones.

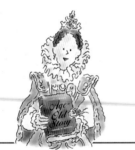

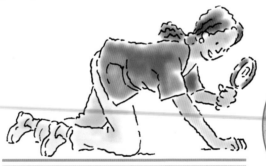

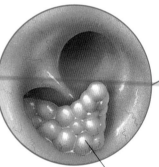

Bronchoscopic view

Tumor projecting into bronchi

Age-old story

Age and lung cancer

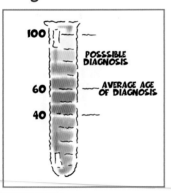

100 — POSSSIBLE DIAGNOSIS

60 — AVERAGE AGE OF DIAGNOSIS

40 —

How it happens

Lung cancer most commonly results from repeated tissue trauma from inhalation of irritants or carcinogens.

Almost all lung cancers start in the epithelium of the lungs. In normal lungs, the epithelium lines and protects the tissue below it. However, when exposed to irritants or carcinogens, the epithelium continually replaces itself until the cells develop chromosomal changes and become dysplastic (altered in size, shape, and organization).

Dysplastic cells don't function well as protectors, so underlying tissue becomes exposed to irritants and carcinogens. Eventually, the dysplastic cells turn into neoplastic carcinoma and start invading deeper tissues.

What to look for

- Cough
- Hoarseness
- Wheezing
- Dyspnea
- Hemoptysis
- Chest pain
- Fever
- Weight loss
- Weakness
- Anorexia
- Dysphagia

Tumor infiltration

Right lung—
anterior view

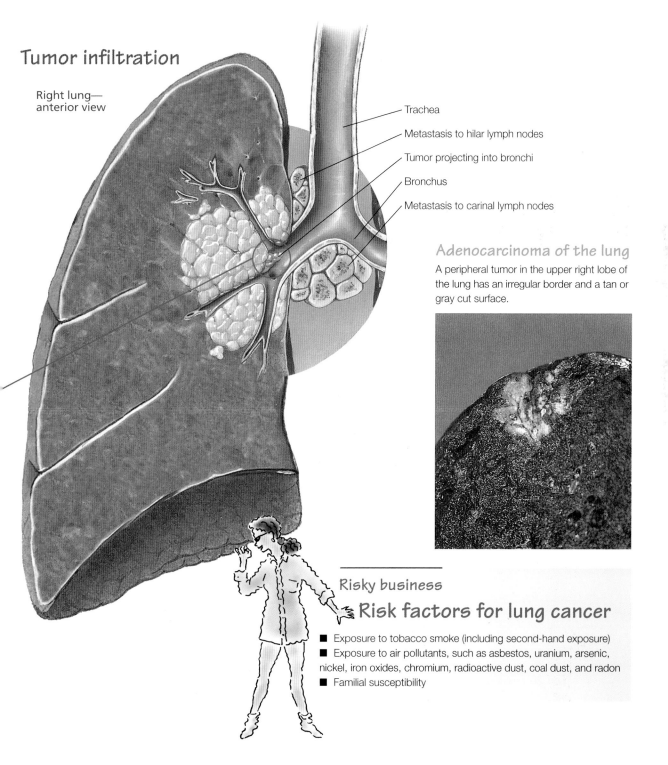

Trachea

Metastasis to hilar lymph nodes

Tumor projecting into bronchi

Bronchus

Metastasis to carinal lymph nodes

Adenocarcinoma of the lung

A peripheral tumor in the upper right lobe of the lung has an irregular border and a tan or gray cut surface.

Risky business
Risk factors for lung cancer

- Exposure to tobacco smoke (including second-hand exposure)
- Exposure to air pollutants, such as asbestos, uranium, arsenic, nickel, iron oxides, chromium, radioactive dust, coal dust, and radon
- Familial susceptibility

Pneumonia

Pneumonia is an acute infection of the lung parenchyma that commonly impairs gas exchange.

It occurs in both genders and at all ages. More than 4 million cases of pneumonia occur annually in the United States. It's the leading cause of death from infectious disease.

The prognosis is good for patients with normal lungs and adequate immune systems. However, bacterial pneumonia is the leading cause of death in debilitated patients.

How it happens

In bacterial pneumonia, an infection triggers alveolar inflammation and edema. This produces an area of low ventilation with normal perfusion. Capillaries become engorged with blood, causing stasis. As the alveolo-capillary membrane breaks down, alveoli fill with blood and exudates, resulting in atelectasis.

In viral pneumonia, the virus attacks bronchial epithelial cells, causing inflammation and desquamation. The virus also invades mucous glands and goblet cells, spreading to the alveoli, which fill with blood and fluid.

Risky business

Risk factors for pneumonia

- Chronic illness and debilitation
- Cancer (particularly lung cancer)
- Abdominal and thoracic surgery
- Atelectasis
- Colds or other viral respiratory infections
- Chronic respiratory disease, such as COPD, bronchiectasis, or cystic fibrosis
- Influenza
- Smoking
- Malnutrition
- Alcoholism
- Sickle cell disease
- Tracheostomy
- Exposure to noxious gases
- Aspiration
- Immunosuppressive therapy
- Premature birth

Classifications

Origin
Pneumonia may be viral, bacterial, fungal, or protozoal in origin.

Location
Bronchopneumonia involves distal airways and alveoli; lobular pneumonia, part of a lobe; and lobar pneumonia, an entire lobe.

Type
Primary pneumonia results from inhalation or aspiration of a pathogen, such as bacteria or a virus, and includes pneumococcal and viral pneumonia; *secondary* pneumonia may follow lung damage from a noxious chemical or other insult or may result from hematogenous spread of bacteria; *aspiration* pneumonia results from inhalation of foreign matter, such as vomitus or food particles, into the bronchi.

Lobar pneumonia

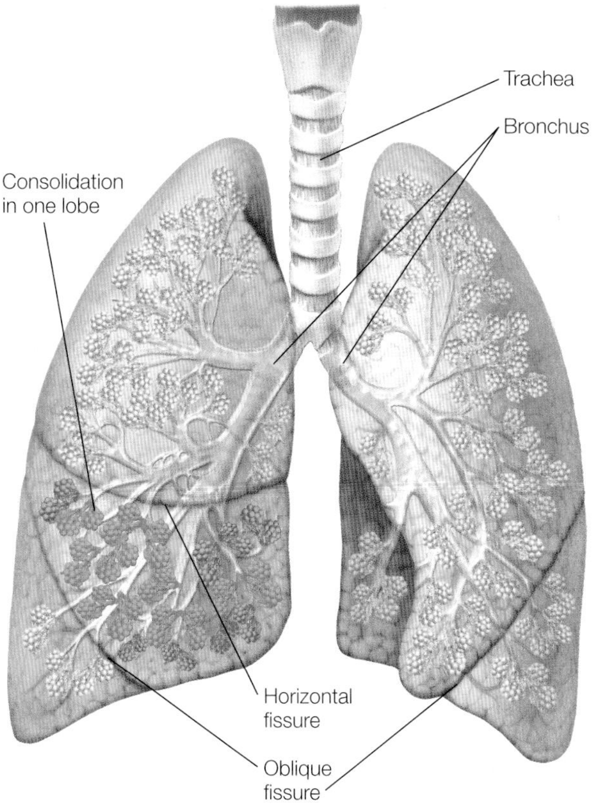

Trachea

Bronchus

Consolidation in one lobe

Horizontal fissure

Oblique fissure

Bronchopneumonia

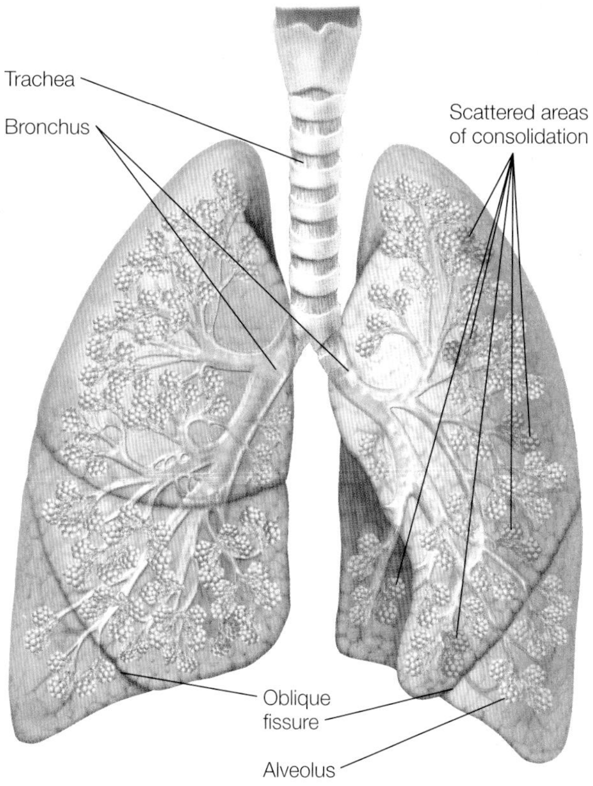

Trachea

Bronchus

Scattered areas of consolidation

Oblique fissure

Alveolus

What to look for

- Fever
- Pleuritic pain
- Chills
- Malaise
- Tachypnea
- Dyspnea
- Cough with purulent, yellow, or bloody sputum
- Crackles
- Decreased breath sounds

Pneumothorax

Pneumothorax is an accumulation of air in the pleural cavity that leads to partial or complete lung collapse. The most common types of pneumothorax are open, closed, and tension.

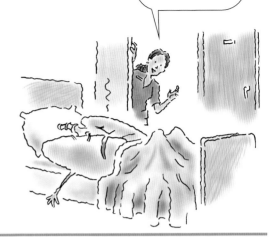

Now that's what I call a collapse!

How it happens

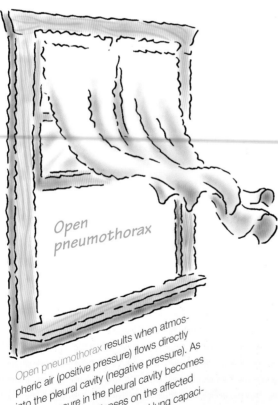

Open pneumothorax

Open pneumothorax results when atmospheric air (positive pressure) flows directly into the pleural cavity (negative pressure). As the air pressure in the pleural cavity becomes positive, the lung collapses on the affected side, resulting in decreased total lung capacity, vital capacity, and lung compliance.

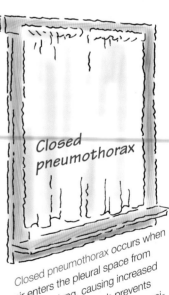

Closed pneumothorax

Closed pneumothorax occurs when air enters the pleural space from within the lung, causing increased pleural pressure, which prevents lung expansion during normal inspiration. Spontaneous pneumothorax is another type of closed pneumothorax.

Open pneumothorax

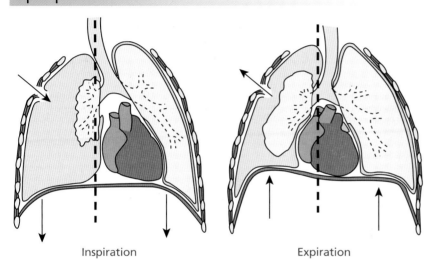

Inspiration   Expiration

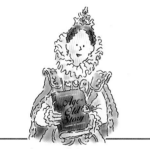

Age-old story

Age and pneumothorax

Spontaneous pneumothorax is common in older patients with chronic pulmonary disease, but it may also occur in healthy, tall young adults.

Closed pneumothorax

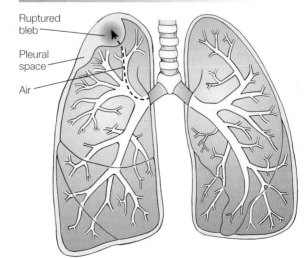

Ruptured bleb

Pleural space

Air

Tension pneumothorax results when air in the pleural space is under higher pressure than air in the adjacent lung. The air enters the pleural space from the site of pleural rupture, which acts as a one-way valve. Air is allowed to enter into the pleural space on inspiration but can't escape as the rupture site closes on expiration. More air enters on inspiration, and air pressure begins to exceed barometric pressure. Increasing air pressure pushes against the recoiled lung, causing compression atelectasis.

As air continues to accumulate and intrapleural pressures increase, the mediastinum shifts away from the affected side and decreases venous return. This forces the heart, trachea, esophagus, and great vessels to the unaffected side, compressing the heart and the contralateral lung.

I'm in high distress. Closed pneumothorax can't be far behind!

What to look for

Closed

- Sudden, sharp, pleuritic pain exacerbated by chest movement, breathing, and coughing
- Asymmetrical chest wall movement
- Shortness of breath
- Cyanosis
- Hyperresonance or tympany heard with percussion
- Respiratory distress

Open

- Signs and symptoms of closed pneumothorax
- Absent breath sounds on the affected side
- Chest rigidity on the affected side
- Tachycardia
- Crackling beneath the skin on palpation

Tension

- Decreased cardiac output
- Hypotension
- Compensatory tachycardia
- Tachypnea
- Lung collapse
- Mediastinal shift and tracheal deviation to the opposite side
- Cardiac arrest

Tension pneumothorax

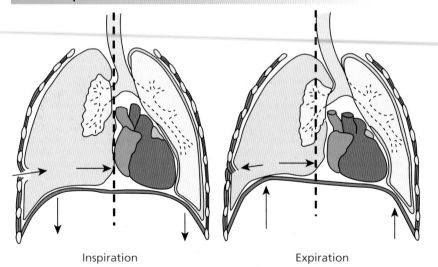

Inspiration

Expiration

Pulmonary edema

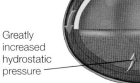

Whoa! This fluid is really accumulating!

Pulmonary edema is a common complication of cardiac disorders. It's marked by accumulated fluid in the extravascular spaces of the lung. It may occur as a chronic condition or develop quickly and rapidly become fatal.

A closer look

Normal

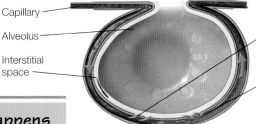

Capillary

Alveolus

Interstitial space

Hydrostatic pressure pushes fluids into the interstitial space.

Plasma oncotic pressure pulls fluids back into the bloodstream.

How it happens

Pulmonary edema may result from left-sided heart failure caused by arteriosclerotic, cardiomyopathic, hypertensive, or valvular heart disease.

Normally, pulmonary capillary hydrostatic pressure, capillary oncotic pressure, capillary permeability, and lymphatic drainage are in balance. This prevents fluid infiltration to the lungs. When this balance changes, or if the lymphatic drainage system is obstructed, pulmonary edema results.

If colloid osmotic pressure decreases, the hydrostatic force that regulates intravascular fluids is lost because nothing opposes it. Fluid flows freely into the interstitium and alveoli, impairing gas exchange and leading to pulmonary edema.

Congestion

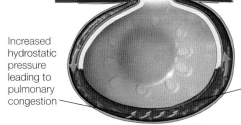

Increased hydrostatic pressure leading to pulmonary congestion

Congested interstitium

Edema

Greatly increased hydrostatic pressure

Large amount of fluid forced into the alveolus

What to look for

Early

- Exertional dyspnea
- Paroxysmal nocturnal dyspnea
- Orthopnea
- Cough
- Mild tachypnea
- Increased blood pressure
- Dependent crackles
- Jugular vein distention
- Tachycardia

Late

- Labored, rapid respiration
- More diffuse crackles
- Cough producing frothy, bloody sputum
- Increased tachycardia
- Arrhythmias
- Cold, clammy skin
- Diaphoresis
- Cyanosis
- Decreased blood pressure
- Thready pulse

Pulmonary embolism

Pulmonary embolism is an obstruction of the pulmonary arterial bed by a dislodged thrombus, heart valve growths, or a foreign substance.

Although pulmonary infarction that results from embolism may be so mild as to produce no symptoms, massive embolism (more than a 50% obstruction of pulmonary arterial circulation) and the accompanying infarction can be rapidly fatal.

How it happens

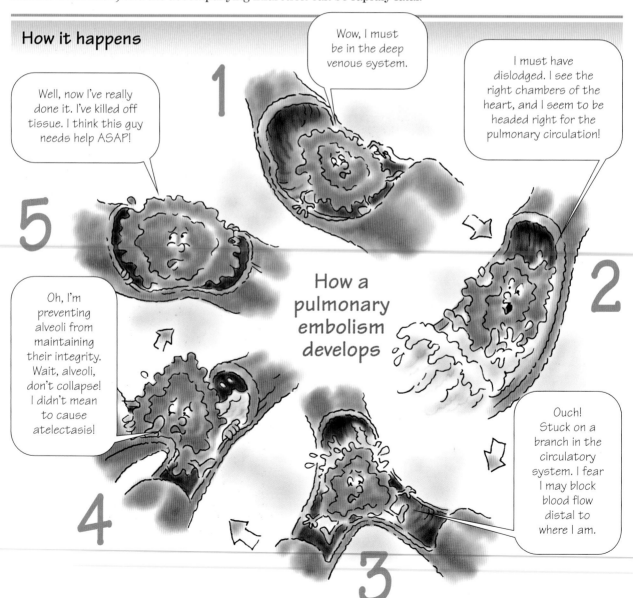

How a pulmonary embolism develops

Pulmonary emboli

What to look for

Common

- Dyspnea
- Anginal or pleuritic chest pain
- Tachycardia
- Productive cough (sputum may be blood-tinged)
- Low-grade fever
- Pleural effusion

Less common

- Massive hemoptysis
- Splinting of the chest
- Leg edema
- Cyanosis
- Syncope
- Distended jugular veins (with a large embolus)
- Pleural friction rub
- Weak, rapid pulse
- Hypotension
- Restlessness
- Anxiety

Infarcted area

Multiple emboli in small branches of left pulmonary artery

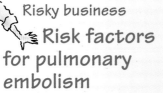

Risky business

Risk factors for pulmonary embolism

- Chronic pulmonary disease
- Heart failure or atrial fibrillation
- Recent surgery
- Thrombophlebitis
- Vascular injury
- Venous stasis
- Varicose veins
- Increased blood coagulability
- Long-term immobility
- Use of hormonal contraceptives
- Obesity

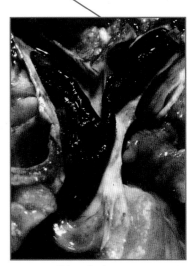

Large, solid embolus

The World Health Organization stated that 8,098 people became ill with SARS during the 2003 outbreak. Of those, 774 died.

Severe acute respiratory syndrome

Severe acute respiratory syndrome (SARS) is a viral respiratory tract infection that can progress to pneumonia and, eventually, death.

The disease was first recognized in 2003 with outbreaks in China, Canada, Singapore, Taiwan, and Vietnam, with other countries—including the United States—reporting smaller numbers of cases. During the 2003 outbreak, SARS was found to be less common among children and to be milder in form in this age-group when it did occur.

How it happens

The SARS virus incubates for 2 to 10 days. The coronavirus that causes SARS is thought to be transmitted by respiratory droplets produced when an infected person coughs or sneezes. The droplets are propelled a short distance (typically up to 3 feet) through the air and deposited on the mucous membranes of the mouth, nose, or eyes of a person who's nearby. The virus can also spread when a person touches a surface or object contaminated with infectious droplets and then touches his mouth, nose, or eyes.

The SARS virion (A) attaches to receptors on the host cell membrane and releases enzymes (called *absorption*) (B) that weaken the membrane and enable the SARS virion to penetrate the cell. The SARS virion removes the protein coating that protects its genetic material (C), replicates (D), and matures, and then escapes from the cell by budding from the plasma membrane (E). The infection then can spread to other host cells.

What to look for

Stage 1
- Fever (greater than 100.4° F [38° C])
- Fatigue
- Headache
- Chills
- Myalgia
- Malaise
- Anorexia
- Diarrhea

Stage 2
- Dry cough
- Dyspnea
- Progressive hypoxemia
- Respiratory failure

Risky business
Risk factors for SARS

- Close contact with an infected person
- Contact with aerosolized (exhaled) droplets and body secretions from an infected person
- Travel to endemic areas

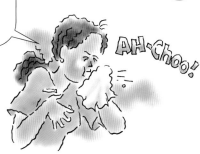

Use tissues to limit those droplets that are responsible for transmitting TB.

AH-Choo!

Tuberculosis

Tuberculosis (TB) is an acute or chronic mycobacterium infection characterized by pulmonary infiltrates and the formation of granulomas with caseation, fibrosis, and cavitation. The main site of infection is the lung, but approximately 15% of infections are extrapulmonary.

How it happens

Multiplication of the bacillus *Mycobacterium tuberculosis* causes an inflammatory process.

A cell-mediated (T-cell) immune response follows that usually contains the infection within 4 to 6 weeks. The T-cell response results in the formation of granulomas around the bacilli, making them dormant. Bacilli within granulomas may remain viable for many years, resulting in a positive purified protein derivative or other skin tests for TB.

Active disease develops in 5% to 15% of those infected with *M. tuberculosis*. Transmission occurs when an infected person coughs or sneezes, which spreads infected droplets.

Primary TB

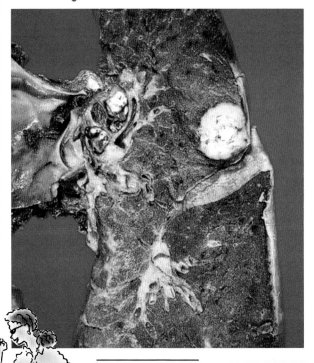

What to look for

- Fatigue
- Cough
- Fever
- Night sweats
- Anorexia
- Weight loss
- Chest pain
- Blood-tinged sputum
- Dullness over the affected area
- Crepitant crackles
- Bronchial breath sounds
- Wheezes
- Whispered pectoriloquy (sound heard through the stethoscope when the patient whispers a word or number)

Risky business
Risk factors for TB

- Close contact with a newly diagnosed patient
- History of previous TB exposure
- Multiple sexual partners
- Recent emigration (from Africa, Asia, Mexico, or South America)
- Gastrectomy
- History of silicosis, diabetes, malnutrition, cancer, Hodgkin's disease, or leukemia
- Drug or alcohol abuse
- Residence in a nursing home, mental health facility, or prison
- Immunosuppression or corticosteroid use
- Homelessness

Upper respiratory tract infection

Upper respiratory tract infection (also known as the *common cold* or *acute coryza*) is an acute, usually afebrile viral infection that causes inflammation of the upper respiratory tract. It's the most common infectious disease. Although a cold is benign and self-limiting, it can lead to secondary bacterial infections.

Well, this looks like as good a place as any to set up camp for a few weeks and see if I can stir up a secondary infection.

How it happens

Infection occurs when the offending organism gains entry into the upper respiratory tract, proliferates, and begins an inflammatory reaction. As a result, acute inflammation of the upper airway structures, including the sinuses, nasopharynx, pharynx, larynx, and trachea, occurs.

The presence of the pathogen triggers infiltration of the mucous membranes by inflammatory and infection-fighting cells. Mucosal swelling and secretion of a serous or mucopurulent exudate result.

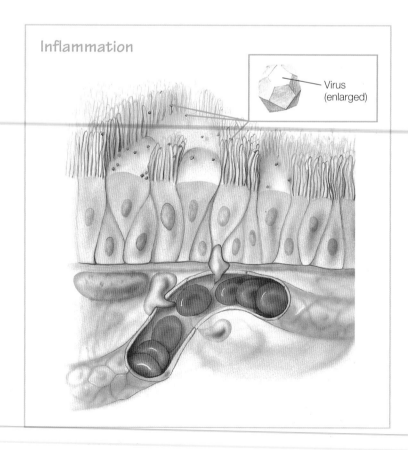

Inflammation

Virus (enlarged)

What to look for

- Pharyngitis
- Nasal congestion
- Coryza (acute rhinitis)
- Sneezing
- Headache
- Burning, watery eyes
- Fever
- Chills
- Myalgia
- Arthralgia
- Malaise
- Lethargy
- Hacking, nonproductive, or nocturnal cough

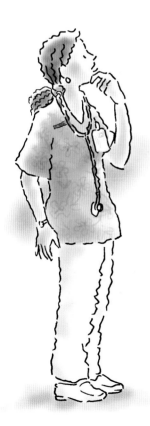

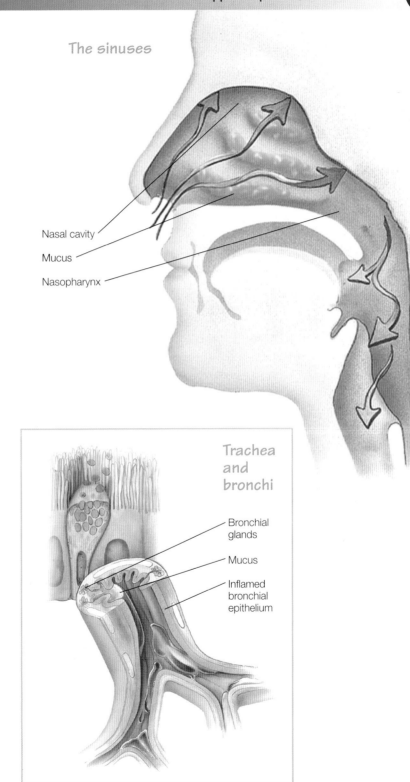

The sinuses

Nasal cavity

Mucus

Nasopharynx

Trachea and bronchi

Bronchial glands

Mucus

Inflamed bronchial epithelium

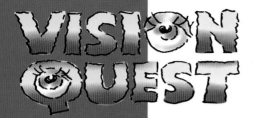

VISION QUEST

My word!

Solve the word scrambles to uncover terms related to respiratory disorders. Then rearrange the circled letters from those words to answer the question posed.

Question: What condition discussed in this chapter is considered to be a chronic obstructive pulmonary disease?

1. horapntomxeu _ _ _ _ _ _ _ ○ ○ _ _ _
2. crisinbhot _ _ _ _ _ _ _ _ _ ○
3. nelaznuif _ _ _ _ _ _ _ _ ○
4. ymseaphme _ ○ _ _ _ _ _ _ ○

Answer: _ _ _ _ _ _

Show and tell

Identify the types of pneumothorax in these illustrations and describe each.

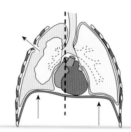

1. ______________________

____

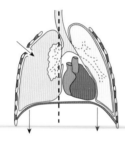

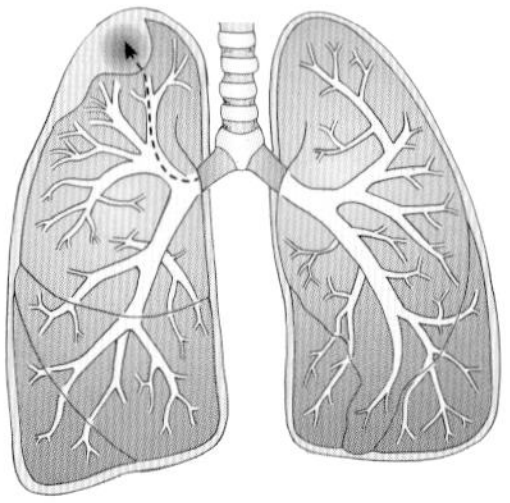

2. ______________________

____

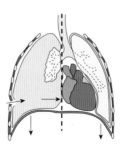

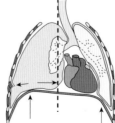

3. ______________________

____

Answers: My word! 1. pneumothorax, 2. bronchitis, 3. influenza, 4. emphysema Question: asthma Show and tell 1. open; occurs when atmospheric air flows directly into the pleural cavity, 2. spontaneous; occurs when air enters the pleural space from within the lung, 3. tension; occurs when air in the pleural space is under higher pressure than air in the adjacent lung.

4 Neurologic disorders

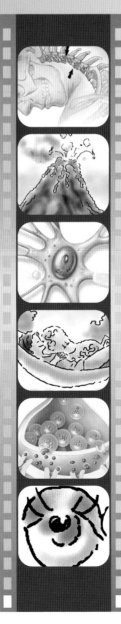

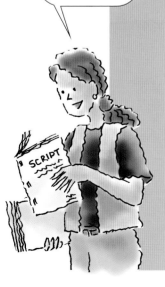

Whiplash, depression, West Nile virus? This chapter has all the makings of a great script.

Acceleration- deceleration cervical injury

Acceleration-deceleration cervical injuries (commonly known as *whiplash*) result from sharp hyperextension and flexion of the neck that damages muscles, ligaments, disks, and nerve tissue. The prognosis for this type of injury is usually excellent; symptoms usually subside when treated.

How it happens

Whiplash injuries of the head and neck

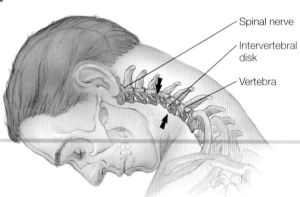

Spinal nerve

Intervertebral disk

Vertebra

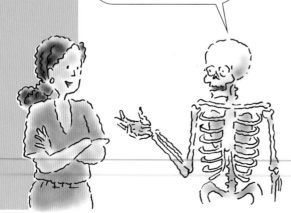

...and all of a sudden, BAM—the guy didn't even slow down. I know it's a cervical injury. I can just feel it!

Hyperflexion

In acceleration-deceleration cervical injuries, the head is propelled in a forward and downward motion in hyperflexion. A wedge-shaped deformity of the bone may be created if the anterior portions of the vertebra are crushed.

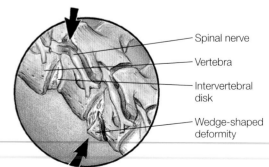

Spinal nerve

Vertebra

Intervertebral disk

Wedge-shaped deformity

What to look for

- Moderate to severe anterior and posterior neck pain
- Dizziness and gait disturbances
- Vomiting
- Headache
- Nuchal rigidity
- Neck muscle asymmetry
- Rigidity or numbness in the arms

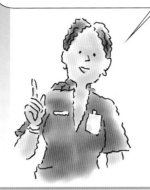

Signs and symptoms may develop immediately or may be completely delayed 12 to 24 hours for mild injury.

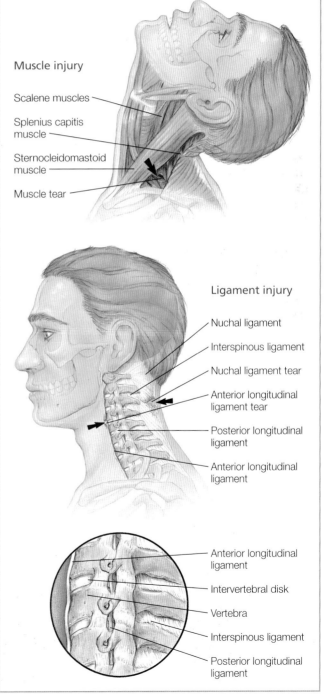

Muscle injury

Scalene muscles

Splenius capitis muscle

Sternocleidomastoid muscle

Muscle tear

Ligament injury

Nuchal ligament

Interspinous ligament

Nuchal ligament tear

Anterior longitudinal ligament tear

Posterior longitudinal ligament

Anterior longitudinal ligament

Anterior longitudinal ligament

Intervertebral disk

Vertebra

Interspinous ligament

Posterior longitudinal ligament

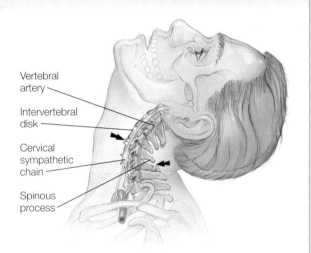

Vertebral artery

Intervertebral disk

Cervical sympathetic chain

Spinous process

Hyperextension

Then the head is forced backward in hyperextension. A tear in the anterior ligament may pull pieces of bone from the cervical vertebrae. Spinous processes of the vertebrae may be fractured. Intervertebral disks may be compressed posteriorly and torn anteriorly. Vertebral arteries may be stretched, pinched, or torn, causing reduced blood flow to the brain. Nerves of the cervical sympathetic chain may also be injured.

Injuries of the neck muscles may range from minor strains and microhemorrhages to severe tears.

Alzheimer's disease

Alzheimer's disease is a progressive, degenerative disorder of the cerebral cortex. Cortical degeneration is most marked in the frontal lobes, but atrophy occurs in all areas of the cortex.

> Because Alzheimer's disease accounts for more than one-half of all dementia cases, I'm trying to keep my mind active!

How it happens

The cause of Alzheimer's disease is unknown, but there are thought to be four contributing factors:

1 neurochemical factors, such as deficiencies in the neuro-transmitters acetylcholine, somatostatin, substance P, and norepinephrine

2 viral factors such as slow-growing central nervous system (CNS) viruses

3 trauma

4 genetic factors.

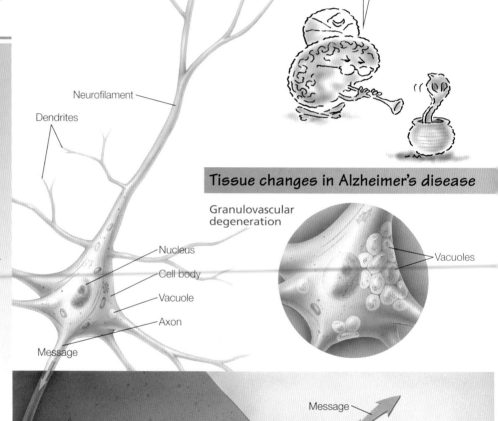

Neurofilament

Dendrites

Nucleus

Cell body

Vacuole

Axon

Message

Tissue changes in Alzheimer's disease

Granulovascular degeneration

Vacuoles

Message

Neurotransmitter (acetylcholine)

Receptor site

Synapse

Granules containing neurotransmitter

Dendrite of receiving neuron

Axon

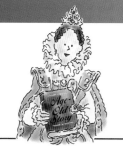

Age-old story

Age and Alzheimer's disease

Although Alzheimer's disease primarily occurs in the elderly population, 1% to 10% of Alzheimer's cases have their onset in middle age.

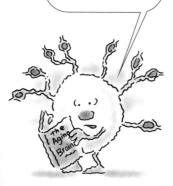

The age of neurons like me seems to play a role in Alzheimer's.

What to look for

Early

- ■ Forgetfulness
- ■ Subtle memory loss without loss of social skills or behavior patterns
- ■ Difficulty learning and retaining new information
- ■ Inability to concentrate
- ■ Deterioration in personal hygiene and appearance

Progressive

- ■ Difficulty with abstract thinking and activities that require judgment
- ■ Progressive difficulty in communicating
- ■ Severe deterioration of memory, language, and motor function progressing to coordination loss and the inability to speak or write
- ■ Repetitive actions
- ■ Restlessness
- ■ Irritability, depression, mood swings, paranoia, hostility, and combativeness
- ■ Nocturnal awakenings
- ■ Disorientation

Neurofibrillar tangles in the neuron

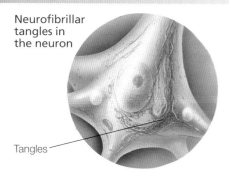

Tangles

Neuritic plaques outside neurons

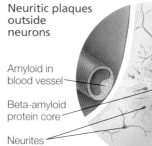

Amyloid in blood vessel

Beta-amyloid protein core

Neurites

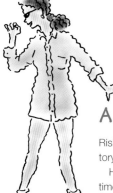

Risky business

Risk factors for Alzheimer's disease

I can't remember whether I'm unable to concentrate because of a disorder or because this feels so good!

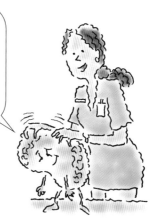

Risk factors for developing Alzheimer's disease are age and a family history of the disease.

Having a parent or a sibling with the disease makes you two to three times more at risk for developing the disease than if you didn't have a parent or sibling with the disease. The more individuals in a family who have the disease, the greater the risk of others in the family developing it.

Cerebral aneurysm

In an intracranial or cerebral aneurysm, a weakness in the wall of the cerebral artery causes localized dilation. Cerebral aneurysms usually arise at an arterial junction in the circle of Willis, the circular anastomosis connecting the major cerebral arteries at the base of the brain. Many cerebral aneurysms rupture, causing a subarachnoid hemorrhage.

> Cerebral aneurysms are generally asymptomatic until they rupture. Look out!

How it happens

Prolonged hemodynamic stress and local arterial degeneration at vessel bifurcations are believed to be major contributing factors in the development and eventual rupture of cerebral aneurysms.

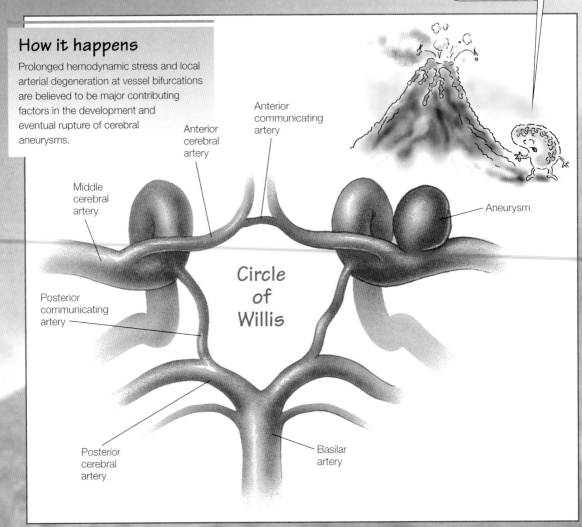

Anterior cerebral artery

Anterior communicating artery

Middle cerebral artery

Aneurysm

Posterior communicating artery

Circle of Willis

Posterior cerebral artery

Basilar artery

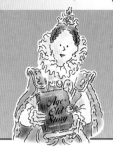

Age and cerebral aneurysm

Incidence is slightly higher in women than in men, especially those in their late 40s or early to mid-50s. However, a cerebral aneurysm may occur at any age and in either gender.

Berry aneurysm

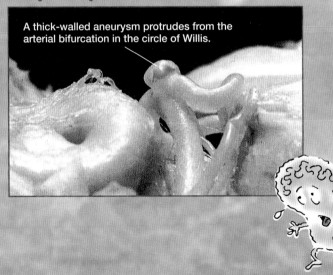

A thick-walled aneurysm protrudes from the arterial bifurcation in the circle of Willis.

What to look for
Subarachnoid hemorrhage
- Change in the level of consciousness
- Sudden severe headache
- Photophobia
- Nuchal rigidity
- Lower back pain
- Nausea and vomiting
- Fever
- Positive Kernig's sign
- Positive Brudzinski's sign
- Seizure
- Cranial nerve deficits
- Motor weakness

Depression

Clinical depression is a serious medical condition that affects thoughts, mood, feelings, behavior, and physical health. It's a persistent condition and can interfere significantly with an individual's ability to function. Clinical depression includes dysthymia, major depression, premenstrual dysmorphic disorder, postpartum depression, and seasonal affective disorder.

The role of neurotransmitters

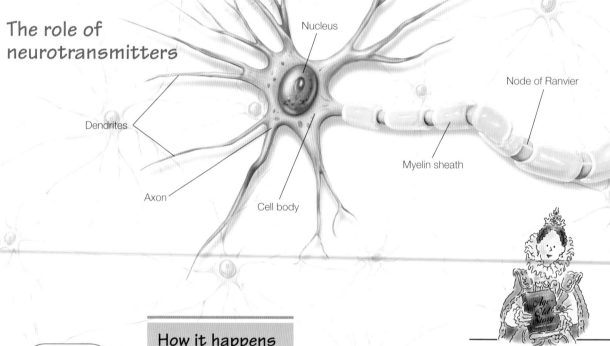

Nucleus

Node of Ranvier

Dendrites

Myelin sheath

Axon

Cell body

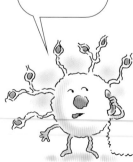

I'd like to send a chemical message, please.

How it happens

Neurotransmitters are chemical messengers released into the synapses (gaps) between neurons that carry messages from one neuron (nerve cell) to another and affect behavior, mood, and thought. Norepinephrine and serotonin are two of the neurotransmitters that play a role in depression. Low levels of these neurotransmitters in areas of the brain that control mood and emotion may result in depression.

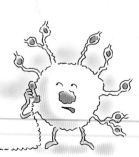

Age-old story

Age and depression

The peak age for the onset of depression is between ages 20 and 40. In children, signs and symptoms of depression include hyperactivity, poor school performance, somatic complaints, sleeping and eating disturbances, lack of playfulness, and suicidal ideation or actions.

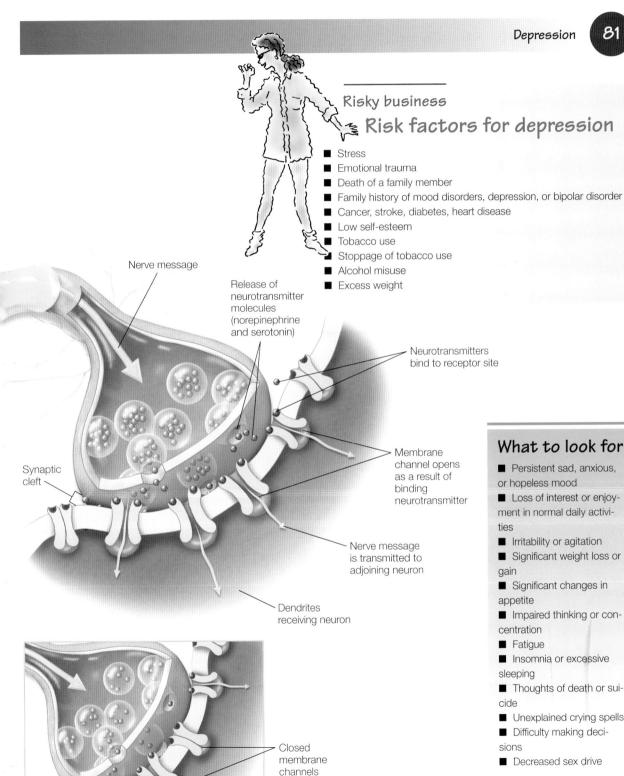

Risky business
Risk factors for depression

- Stress
- Emotional trauma
- Death of a family member
- Family history of mood disorders, depression, or bipolar disorder
- Cancer, stroke, diabetes, heart disease
- Low self-esteem
- Tobacco use
- Stoppage of tobacco use
- Alcohol misuse
- Excess weight

Nerve message

Release of neurotransmitter molecules (norepinephrine and serotonin)

Neurotransmitters bind to receptor site

Membrane channel opens as a result of binding neurotransmitter

Synaptic cleft

Nerve message is transmitted to adjoining neuron

Dendrites receiving neuron

Closed membrane channels

What to look for

- Persistent sad, anxious, or hopeless mood
- Loss of interest or enjoyment in normal daily activities
- Irritability or agitation
- Significant weight loss or gain
- Significant changes in appetite
- Impaired thinking or concentration
- Fatigue
- Insomnia or excessive sleeping
- Thoughts of death or suicide
- Unexplained crying spells
- Difficulty making decisions
- Decreased sex drive

Migraine headache

Migraines can first appear in childhood. Pay attention to the symptoms so you can classify the type.

A migraine headache is a throbbing, vascular headache that usually first appears in childhood and commonly recurs throughout adulthood. It may be classified according to the presence of an aura (temporary focal neurologic signs, usually visual), such as scotoma (an area of lost vision in the visual field), GEOMETRIC SHAPES , JAGGED LINES , ZIGZAG , FLASHING LIGHTS , and colors. A common migraine may not have an aura, whereas a classic migraine has an aura. Migraine headache is more common in women and has a strong familial incidence.

How it happens

Prostaglandin, a hormone present in the bloodstream, signals the platelets to aggregate. Platelet aggregation causes the release of serotonin (a chemical that transmits signals to nerves). Many things can affect the level of serotonin in the body, including blood glucose, certain foods, and changes in estrogen levels.

In a migraine, serotonin levels in the body are increased. This increase in serotonin causes nerves to signal the blood vessels to vasoconstrict or decrease in diameter, which, in turn, causes a decrease in blood flow (ischemia) around the brain. This localized ischemia causes an increase in acid (acidosis). The localized acidosis and ischemia cause noninnervated (no nerves) and innervated blood vessels to dilate.

Vasodilation of the innervated arteries results in the headache phase. Inflammation to the surrounding vessels may prolong the headache pain.

Platelet aggregation then decreases, decreasing the serotonin level, which results in vasodilation. A painful inflammation occurs around the surrounding areas, which can persist.

Theory for the migraine

Normal blood vessel with hormone in bloodstream

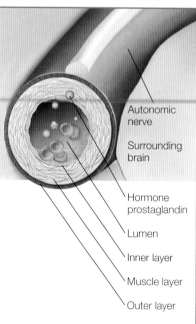

Autonomic nerve

Surrounding brain

Hormone prostaglandin

Lumen

Inner layer

Muscle layer

Outer layer

Constricted blood vessel

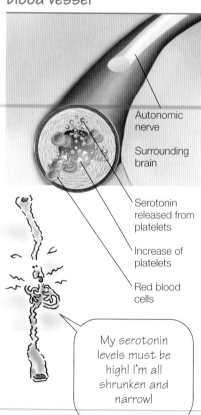

Autonomic nerve

Surrounding brain

Serotonin released from platelets

Increase of platelets

Red blood cells

My serotonin levels must be high! I'm all shrunken and narrow!

The pathways of a migraine

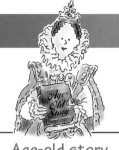

Age-old story

Age and migraines

In children, a common symptom of a migraine headache is intense nausea and vomiting, which may be associated with abdominal pain and fever.

Electrical impulses spread to other regions of the brain.

Chemicals in the brain cause blood vessel dilation and inflammation of surrounding tissue.

Changes in nerve cell activity and blood flow may result in such symptoms as vision disturbances, numbness or tingling, and dizziness.

2

4

3

1

5

Migraine originates deep within the brain.

Dilated blood vessel

Perivascular inflammation from surrounding brain

Decrease of platelets

Red blood cells

Trigeminal nerve ganglion and nuclei

The inflammation irritates the trigeminal nerve, resulting in severe or throbbing pain.

Well, my levels are low. Look how swollen I am! I'm at risk for a migraine!

What to look for

■ Auras
■ Unilateral in onset but may become generalized
■ Begins as a dull ache that progresses into throbbing, pulsating pain
■ Photophobia
■ Nausea and vomiting
■ Paresthesia
■ Phonophobia (fear of sounds)

Multiple sclerosis

Multiple sclerosis (MS) results from progressive demyelination of the white matter of the brain and spinal cord, leading to widespread neurologic dysfunction. The structures usually involved are the optic and oculomotor nerves and the spinal nerve tracts. The disorder doesn't affect the peripheral nervous system. It is characterized by exacerbations and remissions.

How it happens

The exact cause of MS is unknown. It may be due to a slow-acting viral infection, an autoimmune response of the nervous system, or an allergic response. Other possible causes include trauma, anoxia, toxins, nutritional deficiencies, vascular lesions, and anorexia nervosa, all of which may help destroy axons and the myelin sheath.

In addition, emotional stress, overwork, fatigue, pregnancy, or an acute respiratory tract infection may precede the onset of MS. Genetic factors may also play a part.

MS affects the white matter of the brain and spinal cord by creating scattered demyelinated lesions that prevent normal neurologic conduction. After the myelin is destroyed, neuroglial tissue in the white matter of the CNS proliferates, forming hard yellow plaques of scar tissue.

Scar tissue damages the underlying axon fiber, disrupting nerve conduction.

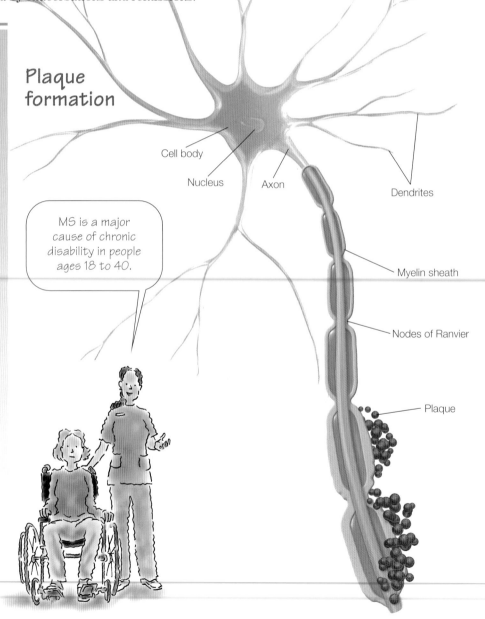

Plaque formation

Cell body

Nucleus

Axon

Dendrites

Myelin sheath

Nodes of Ranvier

Plaque

MS is a major cause of chronic disability in people ages 18 to 40.

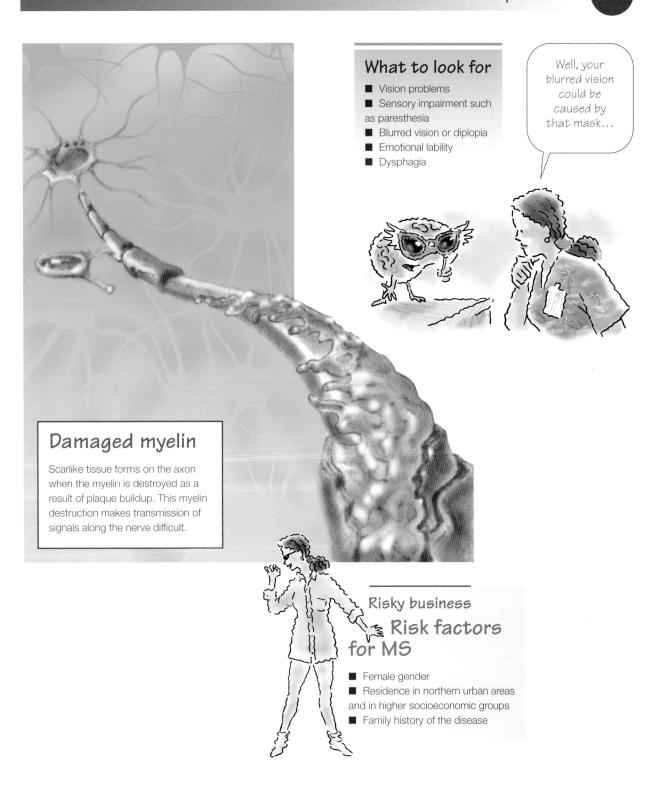

What to look for

- Vision problems
- Sensory impairment such as paresthesia
- Blurred vision or diplopia
- Emotional lability
- Dysphagia

Well, your blurred vision could be caused by that mask...

Damaged myelin

Scarlike tissue forms on the axon when the myelin is destroyed as a result of plaque buildup. This myelin destruction makes transmission of signals along the nerve difficult.

Risky business

Risk factors for MS

- Female gender
- Residence in northern urban areas and in higher socioeconomic groups
- Family history of the disease

Myasthenia gravis

Myasthenia gravis produces sporadic, progressive weakness and abnormal fatigue of voluntary skeletal muscles. These effects are exacerbated by exercise and repeated movement.

Myasthenia gravis usually affects muscles in the face, lips, tongue, neck, and throat, which are innervated by the cranial nerves. However, it can affect any muscle group. Eventually, muscle fibers may degenerate, and weakness (especially of the head, neck, trunk, and limb muscles) may become irreversible. When the disease involves the respiratory system, it may be life-threatening.

I'm tellin' ya, I'm through with exercise. I don't want myasthenia gravis.

I don't think you understand—exercise doesn't cause myasthenia gravis...you just don't want to workout.

How it happens

Normal neuromuscular transmission

Motor nerve impulses travel to motor nerve terminal.

Acetylcholine (ACh) is released.

ACh diffuses across synapse.

ACh receptor sites in motor end plates depolarize muscle fiber.

Depolarization spreads, causing muscle contraction.

Axon

ACh

ACh release site

Normal ACh receptors

Nerve impulses

Motor end plate of muscle

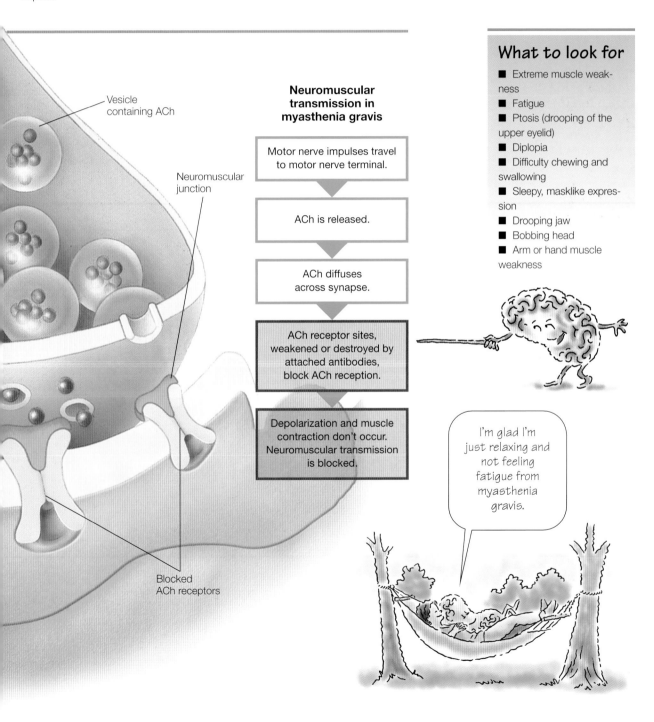

Motor nerve impulse

Vesicle containing ACh

Neuromuscular junction

Blocked ACh receptors

Neuromuscular transmission in myasthenia gravis

Motor nerve impulses travel to motor nerve terminal.

ACh is released.

ACh diffuses across synapse.

ACh receptor sites, weakened or destroyed by attached antibodies, block ACh reception.

Depolarization and muscle contraction don't occur. Neuromuscular transmission is blocked.

What to look for

- Extreme muscle weakness
- Fatigue
- Ptosis (drooping of the upper eyelid)
- Diplopia
- Difficulty chewing and swallowing
- Sleepy, masklike expression
- Drooping jaw
- Bobbing head
- Arm or hand muscle weakness

I'm glad I'm just relaxing and not feeling fatigue from myasthenia gravis.

Parkinson's disease

Parkinson's disease produces progressive muscle rigidity, loss of muscle movement (akinesia), and involuntary tremors. The patient with Parkinson's disease may deteriorate for more than 10 years. Eventually, aspiration pneumonia or some other infection causes death.

Parkinson's disease affects more men than women and usually occurs in middle age or later, striking 1 in every 100 people older than age 60.

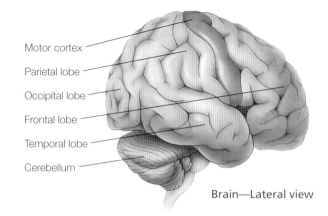

Motor cortex
Parietal lobe
Occipital lobe
Frontal lobe
Temporal lobe
Cerebellum

Brain—Lateral view

How it happens

Parkinson's disease affects the extrapyramidal system, which influences the initiation, modulation, and completion of movement. The extrapyramidal system includes the corpus striatum, globus pallidus, and substantia nigra.

In Parkinson's disease, a dopamine deficiency occurs in the basal ganglia, the dopamine-releasing pathway that connects the substantia nigra to the corpus striatum.

The normal balance upset prevents affected brain cells from performing their normal inhibitory function within the CNS and causes most parkinsonian symptoms.

Neurotransmitter action in Parkinson's disease

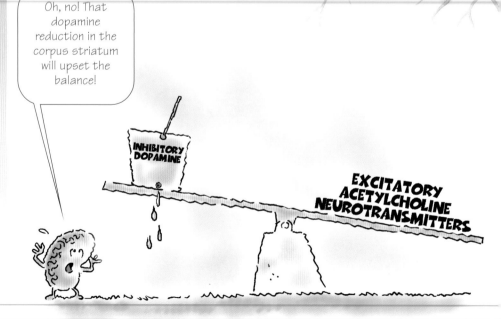

Even though (and maybe because) there are a lot of questions when it comes to Parkinson's disease, it remains one of the most crippling diseases in the United States.

What to look for

- Muscle rigidity, either uniform (lead-pipe rigidity) or jerky (cogwheel rigidity)
- Akinesia
- A unilateral "pill-roll" tremor
- Gait and movement disturbances
- Masklike facial expression
- Blepharospasm (the eyelids stay closed)

Dopamine levels

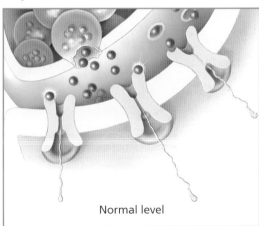

Normal level

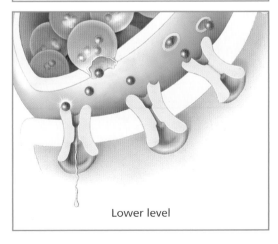

Lower level

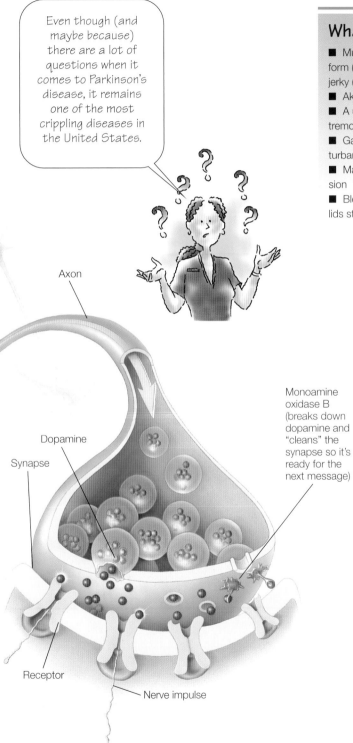

Axon

Dopamine

Synapse

Receptor

Nerve impulse

Monoamine oxidase B (breaks down dopamine and "cleans" the synapse so it's ready for the next message)

Seizure disorder

Seizure disorder (also known as *epilepsy*) is a brain condition characterized by recurrent paroxysmal events associated with abnormal electrical discharges of neurons in the brain. The discharge may trigger a convulsive movement, an interruption of sensation, an alteration in the patient's level of consciousness, or a combination of these symptoms. In most cases, epilepsy doesn't affect intelligence.

It affects people of all ages, races, and ethnic backgrounds; about 2.5 million people have been diagnosed with epilepsy.

How it happens

■ The electronic balance at the neuronal level is altered, causing the membrane of the neuron to become easily activated.

■ Increased permeability of the membranes helps hypersensitive neurons fire abnormally. Abnormal firing may be activated by hyperthermia, hypoglycemia, hyponatremia, hypoxia, or repeated sensory stimulation.

■ When the intensity of a seizure discharge has progressed sufficiently, it spreads to adjacent brain areas. The midbrain, thalamus, and cerebral cortex are most likely to become epileptogenic (producing epileptic attacks).

■ Excitement feeds back from the primary focus and to other parts of the brain.

■ The discharges become less frequent until they stop.

Seizures

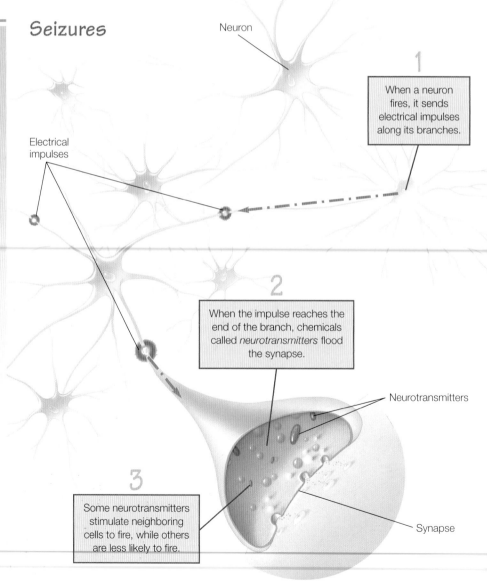

Neuron

Electrical impulses

Neurotransmitters

Synapse

1 When a neuron fires, it sends electrical impulses along its branches.

2 When the impulse reaches the end of the branch, chemicals called *neurotransmitters* flood the synapse.

3 Some neurotransmitters stimulate neighboring cells to fire, while others are less likely to fire.

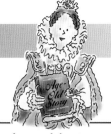

Generalized seizures

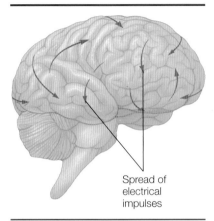

Spread of electrical impulses

Generalized seizures occur as the misfiring signals move across both hemispheres. There's generally no aura, but the patient loses consciousness.

Partial seizures

Complex   Simple

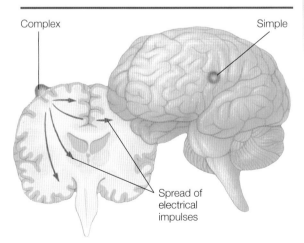

Spread of electrical impulses

A *complex-partial seizure* may begin in one hemisphere, but it quickly moves into both hemispheres. The patient loses consciousness.

A *simple-partial seizure* begins in one hemisphere of the brain. The patient doesn't usually lose consciousness.

Age-old story

Age and seizures

The incidence of seizure disorder is highest in childhood and old age. The prognosis is good if the patient adheres strictly to the prescribed treatment.

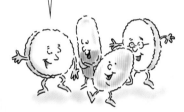

Stick with us, and you'll be in good shape!

What to look for

Auras
- A pungent smell
- Nausea or indigestion
- A rising or sinking feeling in the stomach
- A dreamy feeling
- An unusual taste
- A vision disturbance such as a flashing light

Seizures
- Tonic stiffening followed by muscular contractions
- Tongue biting
- Incontinence
- Blank stare
- Purposeless motor activities
- Changes in level of awareness
- Loss of postural tone
- Jerking and twitching

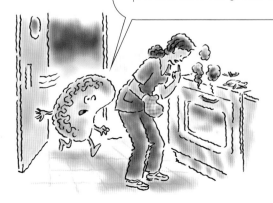

Oh, good—for a minute there I was worried about a seizure. The pungent smell, the sinking feeling in my stomach, and my indigestion were caused by tonight's dinner. The flashing lights were my premonition of the grease fire.

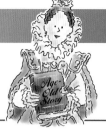

Stroke

A stroke is a sudden impairment of cerebral circulation in one or more of the blood vessels supplying the brain. It interrupts or diminishes oxygen supply, causing serious damage or necrosis in brain tissues. There are two main types:

An ischemic stroke is caused by an interruption of blood flow in a cerebral vessel.

A hemorrhagic stroke is caused by bleeding into the cerebral tissue.

Age-old story

Age and stroke

Although strokes may occur in younger persons, most patients experiencing strokes are older than age 65. In fact, the risk of stroke doubles with each passing decade after age 55.

How it happens

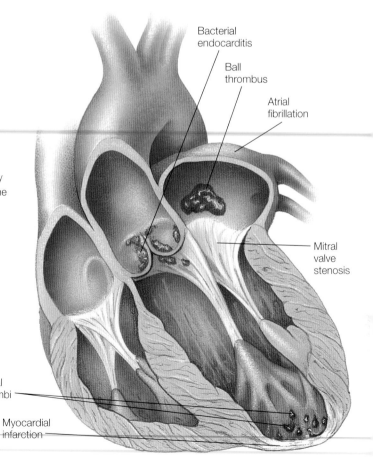

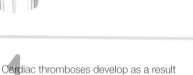

1 Cardiac thromboses develop as a result of various conditions. Emboli break away from their site of origin and move from the heart into the general circulation.

Bacterial endocarditis

Ball thrombus

Atrial fibrillation

Mitral valve stenosis

Mural thrombi

Myocardial infarction

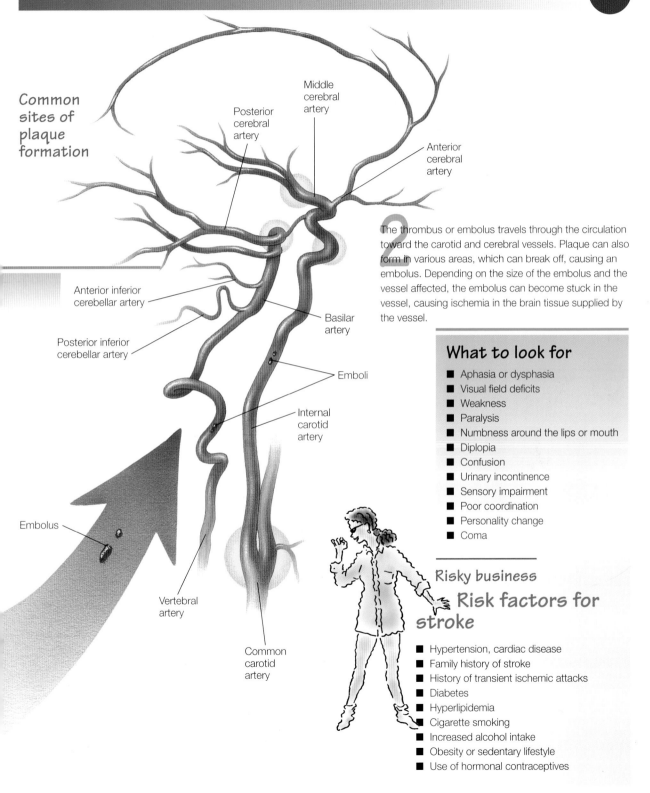

Common sites of plaque formation

Middle cerebral artery

Posterior cerebral artery

Anterior cerebral artery

Anterior inferior cerebellar artery

Posterior inferior cerebellar artery

Basilar artery

Emboli

Internal carotid artery

Embolus

Vertebral artery

Common carotid artery

The thrombus or embolus travels through the circulation toward the carotid and cerebral vessels. Plaque can also form in various areas, which can break off, causing an embolus. Depending on the size of the embolus and the vessel affected, the embolus can become stuck in the vessel, causing ischemia in the brain tissue supplied by the vessel.

What to look for

- Aphasia or dysphasia
- Visual field deficits
- Weakness
- Paralysis
- Numbness around the lips or mouth
- Diplopia
- Confusion
- Urinary incontinence
- Sensory impairment
- Poor coordination
- Personality change
- Coma

Risky business
Risk factors for stroke

- Hypertension, cardiac disease
- Family history of stroke
- History of transient ischemic attacks
- Diabetes
- Hyperlipidemia
- Cigarette smoking
- Increased alcohol intake
- Obesity or sedentary lifestyle
- Use of hormonal contraceptives

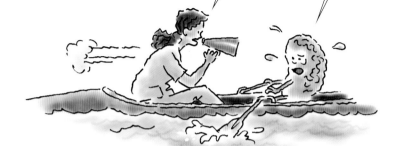

Cerebral hemorrhage

A cerebral hemorrhage can occur like this one, which produced a hematoma that extended into the ventricle, almost rupturing it.

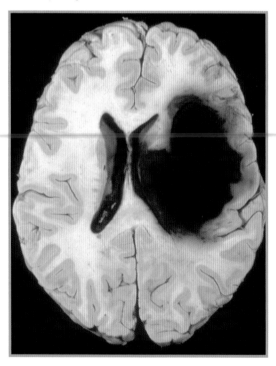

Subarachnoid hemorrhage

Hypertension may cause microaneurysms and tiny arterioles to rupture in the brain, creating pressure on adjacent arterioles and causing them to burst, which leads to more bleeding. Trauma can cause a subarachnoid hemorrhage, which places more pressure on brain tissue.

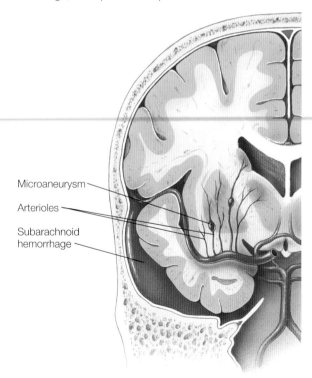

Microaneurysm

Arterioles

Subarachnoid hemorrhage

West Nile encephalitis

West Nile encephalitis is a vector-borne disease that primarily results in encephalitis (inflammation) of the brain. It's caused by the West Nile virus, a flavivirus (the type of mosquito- or tickborne virus responsible for yellow fever and malaria) commonly found in humans, birds, and other vertebrates.

How it happens

Humans are believed to be the "dead-end-hosts"—the virus lives in people and can make them ill, but feeding mosquitos can't acquire the virus from biting an infected person. After the pathogen enters the bloodstream, it travels to the brain and causes encephalitis.

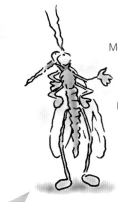

Mosquitos serve as the vectors, spreading the virus from bird to bird and from birds to people.

Birds harbor the West Nile virus but can't spread it on their own.

memory board

To remember the key signs and symptoms of West Nile encephalitis, think FRESH:

Fever

Rashes

Extreme fatigue

Swollen lymph glands

Head and body aches.

Think *fresh*, then think about spring: springtime is the start of the West Nile season.

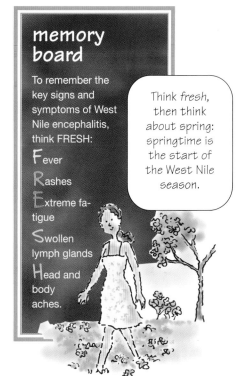

What to look for

- Fever
- Extreme fatigue
- Head and body aches
- Rashes
- Swollen lymph glands

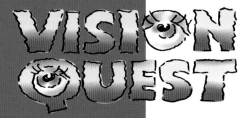

Matchmaker

Match the whiplash injury with its correct name.

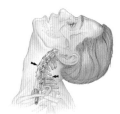 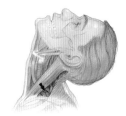 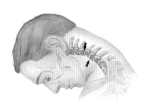

1. _____   2. _____   3. _____

A. muscle injury
B. hyperflexion
C. hyperextension

Able to label?

In the illustration, label the brain structures.

1. _____
2. _____
3. _____
4. _____
5. _____
6. _____

5 Gastrointestinal disorders

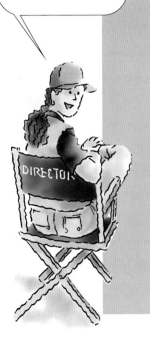

OK, everyone. Let's break for lunch! And try not to upset your GI system this time.

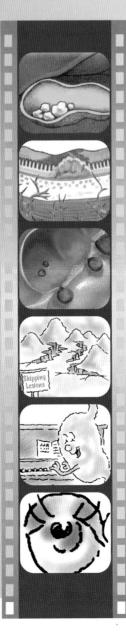

Skipping Lesions

DIRECTOR

Cholecystitis

In cholecystitis, the gallbladder becomes inflamed. Usually, a calculus (gallstone) becomes lodged in the cystic duct, causing painful gallbladder distention. Cholecystitis may be acute or chronic.

Understanding gallstone formation

Abnormal metabolism of cholesterol and bile salts plays an important role in gallstone formation. The liver makes bile continuously. The gallbladder concentrates and stores it until the duodenum signals it needs bile to help digest fat. Changes in the composition of bile may allow gallstones to form. Changes to the absorptive ability of the gallbladder lining may also contribute to gallstone formation.

Inside the liver

Certain conditions, such as age, obesity, and estrogen imbalance, cause the liver to secrete bile that's abnormally high in cholesterol or lacking the proper concentration of bile salts.

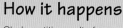

Cholesterol metabolism and bile salts seem to be main culprits at this point.

How it happens

Cholecystitis results from the formation of gallstones. The exact cause of gall-stone formation is un-known but it's thought that abnormal metabolism of cholesterol and bile salts plays an important role. Acute cholecystitis may also be due to poor or ab-sent blood flow to the gall-bladder.

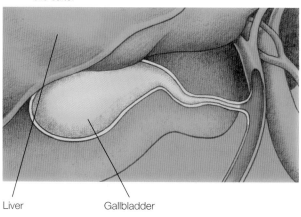

Liver　　　　　Gallbladder

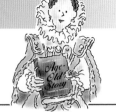

Inside the gallbladder

When the gallbladder concentrates this bile, inflammation may occur. Excessive reabsorption of water and bile salts makes the bile less soluble. Cholesterol, calcium, and bilirubin precipitate into gallstones.

Fat entering the duodenum causes the intestinal mucosa to secrete the hormone cholecystokinin, which stimulates the gallbladder to contract and empty. If a stone lodges in the cystic duct, the gallbladder contracts but can't empty.

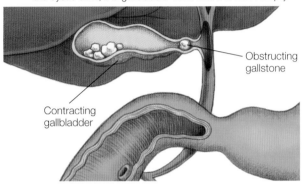

Obstructing gallstone

Contracting gallbladder

Inside the common bile duct

If a stone lodges in the common bile duct, the bile can't flow into the duodenum. Bilirubin is absorbed into the blood and causes jaundice.

Biliary narrowing and swelling of the tissue around the stone can also cause irritation and inflammation of the common bile duct.

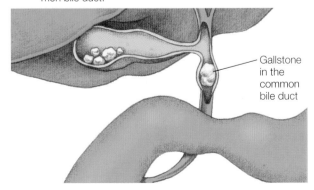

Gallstone in the common bile duct

Inside the biliary tree

Inflammation can progress up the biliary tree into any of the bile ducts. This causes scar tissue, fluid accumulation, cirrhosis, portal hypertension, and bleeding.

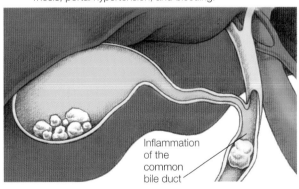

Inflammation of the common bile duct

What to look for

- Acute abdominal pain in the right upper quadrant that may radiate to the back, between the shoulders, or to the front of the chest
- Colic
- Nausea and vomiting
- Chills
- Low-grade fever
- Jaundice
- Belching
- Flatulence
- Indigestion
- Light-headedness

Cirrhosis

Cirrhosis, a chronic liver disease, is characterized by widespread destruction of hepatic cells, which are replaced by fibrous cells through a process called *fibrotic regeneration*.

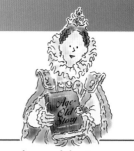

Age and cirrhosis

Cirrhosis is especially prevalent among malnourished people older than age 50 with chronic alcoholism; it's also twice as common in men as in women.

How it happens

The changes that occur in cirrhosis, such as irreversible chronic injury of the liver, extensive fibrosis, and nodular tissue growth, result from liver cell death, collapse of the liver's supporting structure, distortion of the vascular bed, and nodular regeneration of remaining liver tissue.

Most cases are a result of alcoholism, but toxins, biliary destruction, hepatitis, and a number of metabolic conditions may stimulate the destruction process.

There are many types of cirrhosis; causes differ with each type and include the following:

■ Laënnec's cirrhosis—also called *portal, nutritional,* or *alcoholic cirrhosis*—is the most common type and is commonly caused by hepatitis C. Liver damage results from malnutrition (especially dietary protein) and overuse of alcohol.

■ Biliary cirrhosis results from bile duct diseases suppressing bile flow.

■ Pigment cirrhosis may result from bile duct diseases, such as Wilson's disease, alpha$_1$-antitrypsin deficiency, and hemochromatosis.

■ Other types of cirrhosis include Budd-Chiari syndrome, cardiac cirrhosis, and cryptogenic cirrhosis. Cardiac cirrhosis is rare; the liver damage results from right-sided heart failure. Cryptogenic refers to cirrhosis of unknown cause.

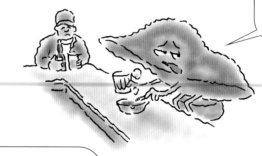

Alcohol is not a friend, especially if the person is male and middle-aged.

Nutrition plays a role in nutritional cirrhosis. This spread would have done a cirrhosis patient some good!

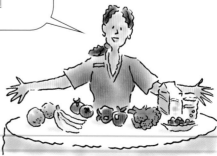

Cirrhosis of the liver

The surface of the liver shows small nodules as opposed to the normally smooth surface.

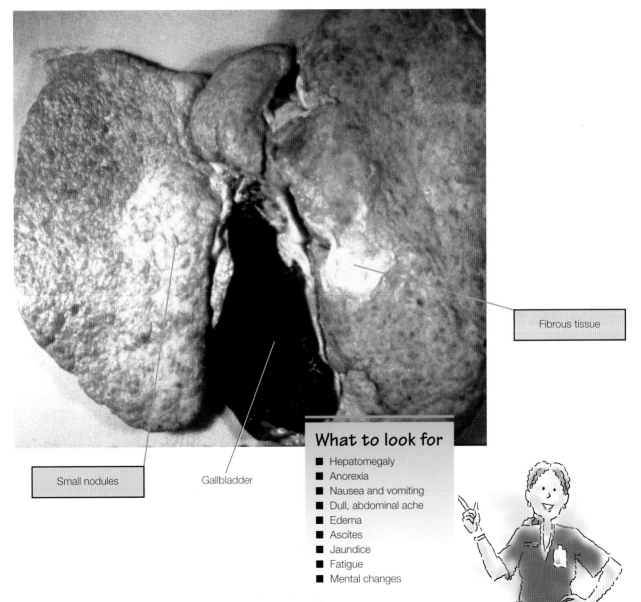

Fibrous tissue

Small nodules

Gallbladder

What to look for

- Hepatomegaly
- Anorexia
- Nausea and vomiting
- Dull, abdominal ache
- Edema
- Ascites
- Jaundice
- Fatigue
- Mental changes

Colorectal cancer

Colorectal cancer is a slow-growing adenocarcinoma that usually starts in the inner layer of the intestinal tract. It commonly begins as a polyp and is potentially curable if diagnosed early.

How it happens

The exact cause of colorectal cancer is unknown. Bacteria have been associated with the conversion of bile acids into carcinogens, and a diet high in refined sugar aids in this process.

Types of colorectal cancer

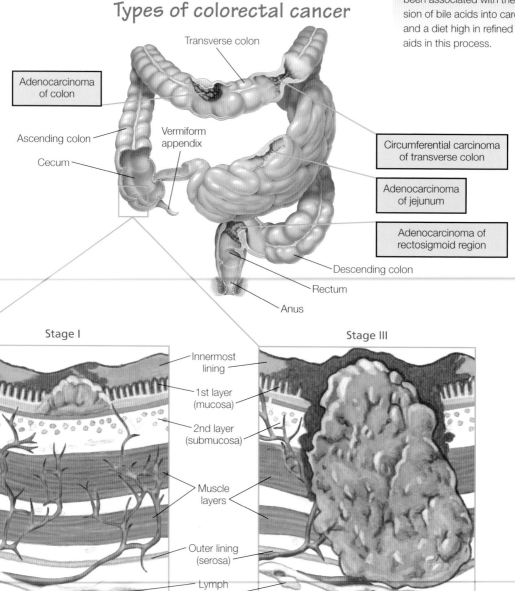

Transverse colon

Adenocarcinoma of colon

Ascending colon

Vermiform appendix

Cecum

Circumferential carcinoma of transverse colon

Adenocarcinoma of jejunum

Adenocarcinoma of rectosigmoid region

Descending colon

Rectum

Anus

Stage I

Stage III

Innermost lining

1st layer (mucosa)

2nd layer (submucosa)

Muscle layers

Outer lining (serosa)

Lymph nodes

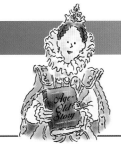

Age and colorectal cancer

Being older than age 40 is a risk factor for colorectal cancer.

What to look for

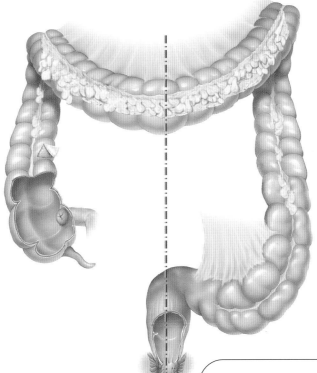

On the right

- Black, tarry stools
- Rectal bleeding
- Anemia
- Abdominal aching, pressure, or dull cramps
- Weakness
- Fatigue
- Exertional dyspnea
- Diarrhea
- Obstipation
- Anorexia
- Weight loss
- Vomiting

On the left

- Black, tarry stools or rectal bleeding
- Intermittent abdominal fullness or cramping; rectal pressure
- Obstipation
- Diarrhea or "ribbonlike" stool
- Dark or bright red blood in stool; mucus in or on stool

Risky business

Risk factors for colorectal cancer

- Inherited gene mutations
- Family or personal history of colorectal cancer, Crohn's disease, or ulcerative colitis
- History of intestinal polyps
- Aging
- High-fat diet
- Obesity and physical inactivity
- Diabetes
- Smoking
- Heavy alcohol intake

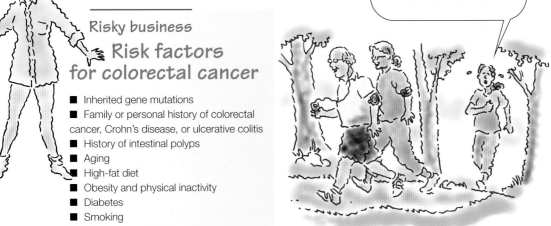

I'm glad all I inherited was my love of jogging. How much further??

Crohn's disease

Crohn's disease is one of two major types of inflammatory bowel disease. It may affect any part of the GI tract. Inflammation extends through all layers of the intestinal wall and may involve lymph nodes and supporting membranes in the area. Ulcers form as the inflammation extends into the peritoneum. Crohn's disease is most prevalent in adults ages 20 to 40.

Crohn's disease affects men and women equally. It also tends to run in families—up to 20% of patients with the disease have a history of it in their family.

How it happens

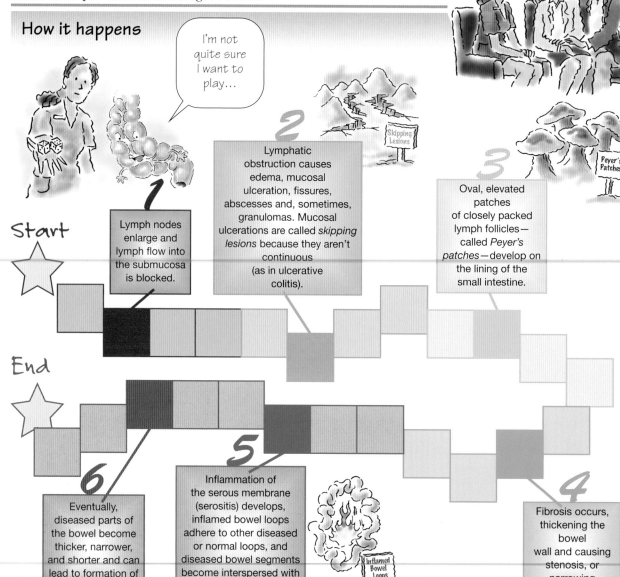

I'm not quite sure I want to play...

Start

1 Lymph nodes enlarge and lymph flow into the submucosa is blocked.

2 Lymphatic obstruction causes edema, mucosal ulceration, fissures, abscesses and, sometimes, granulomas. Mucosal ulcerations are called *skipping lesions* because they aren't continuous (as in ulcerative colitis).

Skipping Lesions

3 Oval, elevated patches of closely packed lymph follicles—called *Peyer's patches*—develop on the lining of the small intestine.

Peyer's Patches

End

6 Eventually, diseased parts of the bowel become thicker, narrower, and shorter and can lead to formation of strictures.

5 Inflammation of the serous membrane (serositis) develops, inflamed bowel loops adhere to other diseased or normal loops, and diseased bowel segments become interspersed with healthy ones.

Inflamed Bowel Loops

4 Fibrosis occurs, thickening the bowel wall and causing stenosis, or narrowing of the lumen.

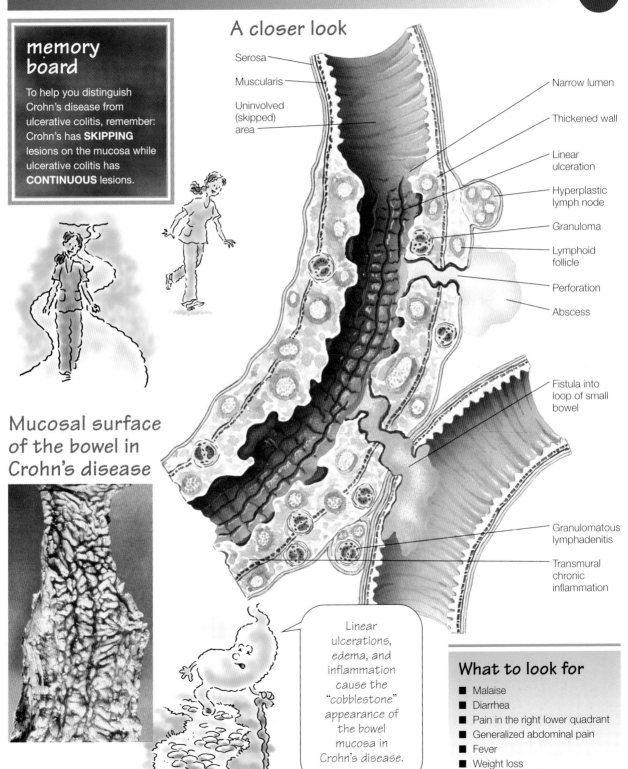

memory board

To help you distinguish Crohn's disease from ulcerative colitis, remember: Crohn's has **SKIPPING** lesions on the mucosa while ulcerative colitis has **CONTINUOUS** lesions.

A closer look

Serosa

Muscularis

Uninvolved (skipped) area

Narrow lumen

Thickened wall

Linear ulceration

Hyperplastic lymph node

Granuloma

Lymphoid follicle

Perforation

Abscess

Fistula into loop of small bowel

Granulomatous lymphadenitis

Transmural chronic inflammation

Mucosal surface of the bowel in Crohn's disease

Linear ulcerations, edema, and inflammation cause the "cobblestone" appearance of the bowel mucosa in Crohn's disease.

What to look for

- Malaise
- Diarrhea
- Pain in the right lower quadrant
- Generalized abdominal pain
- Fever
- Weight loss

Diverticular disease

In diverticular disease, bulging, pouchlike herniations (diverticula) in the GI wall push the mucosal lining through the surrounding muscle. Diverticula occur most commonly in the sigmoid colon, but they may develop anywhere, from the proximal end of the pharynx to the anus.

Diverticular disease has two clinical forms:

1 diverticulosis—diverticula are present but produce no symptoms

2 diverticulitis—inflamed diverticula that may cause potentially fatal obstruction, infection, and hemorrhage.

> Location is everything in real estate. Diverticular disease can occur anywhere along the digestive tract but it's most common on the left side of the colon.

How it happens

Diverticula probably result from high intraluminal pressure on an area of weakness in the GI wall where blood vessels enter. Diet may be a contributing factor because insufficient fiber reduces fecal residue, narrows the bowel lumen, and leads to high intra-abdominal pressure during defecation.

In diverticulitis, retained undigested food and bacteria accumulate in the diverticular sac. This hard mass cuts off the blood supply to the thin walls of the sac, making them more susceptible to attack by colonic bacteria. Inflammation follows and may lead to perforation, abscess, peritonitis, obstruction, or hemorrhage. Occasionally, the inflamed colon segment may adhere to the bladder or other organs and cause a fistula.

Diverticulosis of the colon

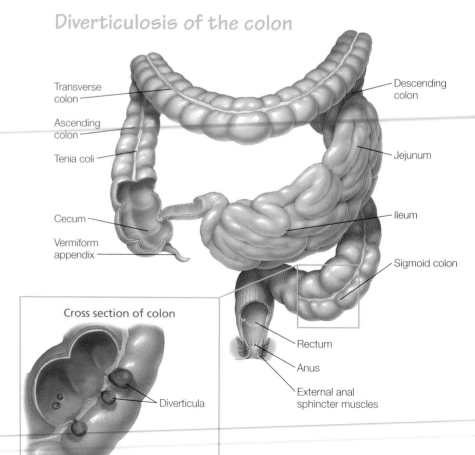

Transverse colon

Descending colon

Ascending colon

Jejunum

Tenia coli

Cecum

Ileum

Vermiform appendix

Sigmoid colon

Cross section of colon

Rectum

Anus

Diverticula

External anal sphincter muscles

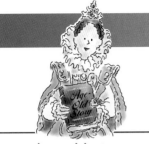

Age-old story

Age and diverticular disease

Diverticular disease is most prevalent in men older than age 40 and in people who eat a low-fiber diet. More than one-half of all people older than age 50 have colonic diverticula.

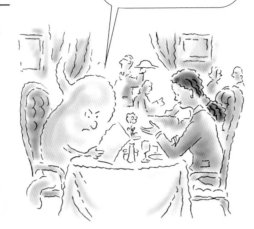

I hate having to watch my diet because of this diverticulitis. I tell you, it isn't fair!

Diverticulosis

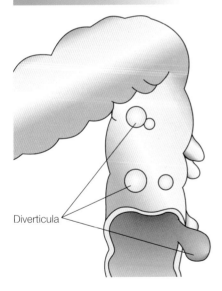

Diverticula

Diverticulitis

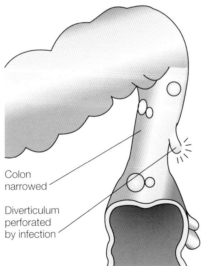

Colon narrowed

Diverticulum perforated by infection

What to look for

Typically the patient with diverticulosis is asymptomatic and will remain so unless diverticulitis develops.

Mild
- Moderate left-sided lower abdominal pain
- Low-grade fever

Severe
- Abdominal rigidity
- Left lower quadrant pain
- High fever
- Chills
- Hypotension

Chronic
- Constipation
- Ribbonlike stools
- Intermittent diarrhea
- Abdominal distention
- Abdominal rigidity and pain
- Diminishing or absent bowel sounds
- Nausea
- Vomiting

Esophageal varices

Esophageal varices are dilated torturous veins in the submucosa of the lower esophagus. In many patients, they're the first sign of portal hypertension (elevated pressure in the portal vein). Esophageal varices commonly cause massive hematemesis (vomiting of blood), requiring emergency care to control hemorrhage and prevent hypovolemic shock.

> Esophageal varices can require emergency care if massive hemorrhage occurs.

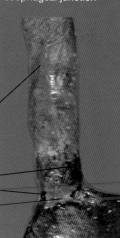

How it happens

Portal hypertension occurs when blood meets increased resistance. As pressure in the portal vein increases, blood backs up into the spleen and flows through collateral channels to the venous system, bypassing the liver.

Esophageal varices have two main inflows—the left gastric or coronary vein and the splenic hilus, through the short gastric veins. These collateral veins become dilated and eventually hemorrhage; esophageal varices are very susceptible to bleeding and hemorrhage.

> I get totally passed by when portal hypertension occurs. Bad news for the esophagus.

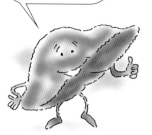

Increased pressure stimulates the development of collateral channels (varices), which attempt to bypass the portal vein flow into the liver.

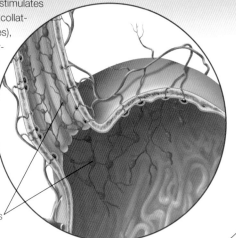

Esophageal and gastric varices

Numerous prominent blue venous channels are seen beneath the mucosa of the everted esophagus, particularly above the gastroesophageal junction

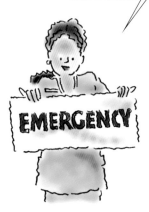

Everted esophagus

Venous channels

Gastroesophageal junction

What happens in portal hypertension

Portal hypertension (elevated pressure in the portal vein) occurs when blood flow meets increased resistance. This common result of cirrhosis may also stem from mechanical obstruction and occlusion of the hepatic veins (Budd-Chiari syndrome).

As the pressure in the portal vein rises, blood backs up into the spleen and flows through collateral channels to the venous system, bypassing the liver. Thus, portal hypertension causes:

■ splenomegaly with thrombocytopenia
■ dilated collateral veins (esophageal varices, hemorrhoids, or prominent abdominal veins)
■ ascites.

In many patients, the first sign of portal hypertension is bleeding esophageal varices (dilated tortuous veins in the submucosa of the lower esophagus).

Esophageal varices commonly cause massive hematemesis, requiring emergency care to control hemorrhage and prevent hypovolemic shock.

As pressure in the portal vein rises, blood backs up into spleen

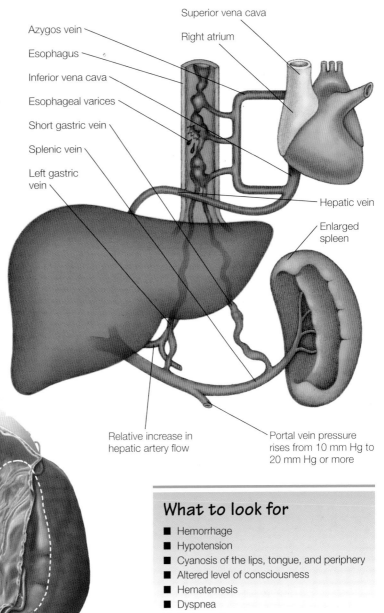

Superior vena cava
Azygos vein
Right atrium
Esophagus
Inferior vena cava
Esophageal varices
Short gastric vein
Splenic vein
Left gastric vein
Hepatic vein
Enlarged spleen

Relative increase in hepatic artery flow

Portal vein pressure rises from 10 mm Hg to 20 mm Hg or more

Size of normal spleen

Splenomegaly (enlargement of spleen)

What to look for

■ Hemorrhage
■ Hypotension
■ Cyanosis of the lips, tongue, and periphery
■ Altered level of consciousness
■ Hematemesis
■ Dyspnea
■ Tachycardia

Gastroesophageal reflux disease

Popularly known as *heartburn*, gastroesophageal reflux disease (GERD) refers to the backflow of gastric and duodenal contents past the lower esophageal sphincter (LES) and into the esophagus without associated belching or vomiting. The reflux of gastric contents causes acute epigastric pain, usually after a meal. The pain may radiate to the chest or arms.

I probably shouldn't have had that extra helping of pasta. The sauce was pretty garlicky...

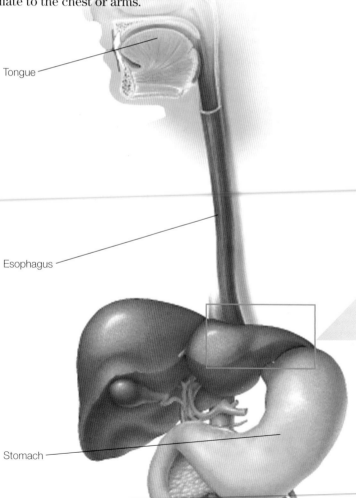

Tongue

Esophagus

Stomach

What to look for

■ Burning pain in the epigastric area, possibly radiating to the arms and chest
■ Pain, usually after a meal or when lying down
■ Feeling of fluid accumulation in the throat without a sour or bitter taste

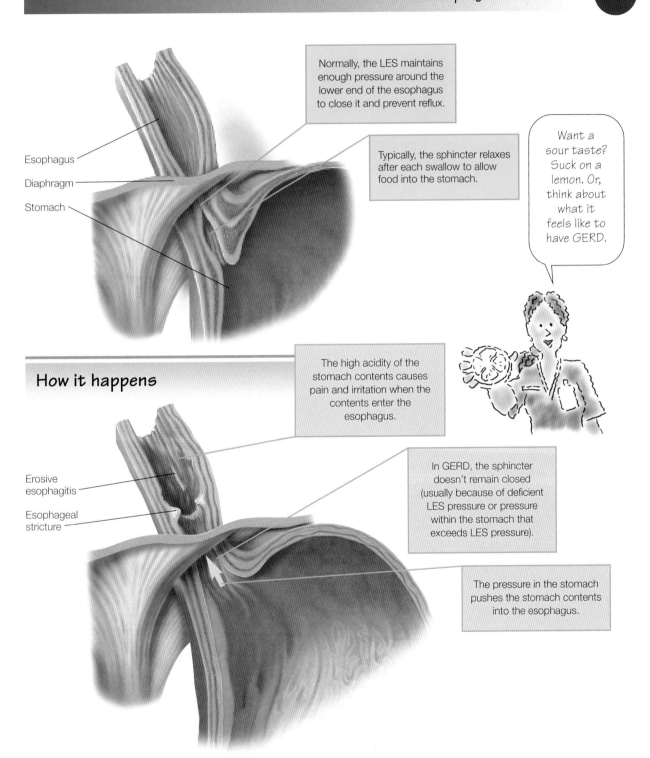

Esophagus

Diaphragm

Stomach

Normally, the LES maintains enough pressure around the lower end of the esophagus to close it and prevent reflux.

Typically, the sphincter relaxes after each swallow to allow food into the stomach.

Want a sour taste? Suck on a lemon. Or, think about what it feels like to have GERD.

How it happens

The high acidity of the stomach contents causes pain and irritation when the contents enter the esophagus.

Erosive esophagitis

Esophageal stricture

In GERD, the sphincter doesn't remain closed (usually because of deficient LES pressure or pressure within the stomach that exceeds LES pressure).

The pressure in the stomach pushes the stomach contents into the esophagus.

Hepatitis, viral

Viral hepatitis is a common infection of the liver. In most patients, liver cells (hepatocytes) damaged by hepatitis eventually regenerate with little or no permanent damage. However, old age and serious underlying disorders make complications more likely.

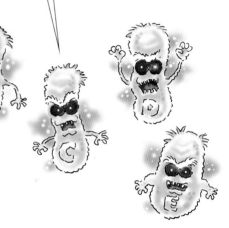

We're the five types of hepatitis!

How it happens

The virus causes hepatocyte injury and death, either by directly killing the cells or by activating inflammatory and immune reactions. The inflammatory and immune reactions, in turn, injure or destroy hepatocytes by causing the infected or neighboring cells to disintegrate. Later, direct antibody attack against the viral antigens causes further destruction of the infected cells. Edema and swelling of the interstitium lead to collapse of capillaries, decreased blood flow, tissue hypoxia, scarring, and fibrosis.

Liver with the effects of hepatitis

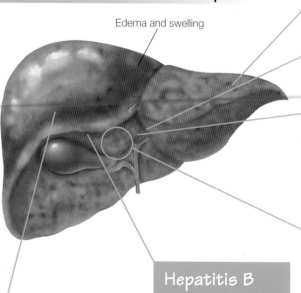

Edema and swelling

Normal liver

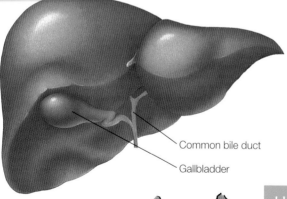

Common bile duct

Gallbladder

Hepatitis A

Highly contagious; results from ingestion of contaminated food or water

Hepatitis B

Blood-borne—parenteral route, sexual, maternal-neonatal; virus is shed in all body fluids

What to look for

Prodromal stage
- Fatigue
- Malaise
- Arthralgia
- Myalgia
- Fever
- Mild weight loss
- Nausea and vomiting
- Changes in senses of taste and smell
- Right upper quadrant tenderness
- Dark-colored urine
- Clay-colored stools

Clinical or icteric stage
- Itching
- Jaundice
- Abdominal pain or tenderness

Recovery stage
- Subsiding symptoms
- Return of appetite

Hepatitis E

Associated with recent travel to endemic areas such as India, Africa, Asia, or Central America; fecal oral route

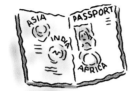

Hepatitis D

Linked to chronic hepatitis B infection

Hepatitis C

Blood-borne: parenteral route associated with shared needles, blood transfusions but it can also be transmitted sexually or by mother to her fetus

Moderate hepatitis

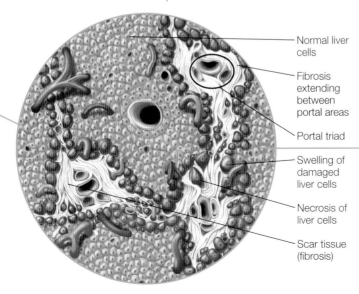

- Normal liver cells
- Fibrosis extending between portal areas
- Portal triad
- Swelling of damaged liver cells
- Necrosis of liver cells
- Scar tissue (fibrosis)

Necrotic liver

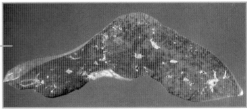

A necrotic liver becomes soft and smaller in size than a normal liver.

Intestinal obstruction

A bowel free from obstruction is music to my ears!

Intestinal obstruction is the partial or complete blockage of the lumen in the small or large bowel. Small-bowel obstruction is far more common and usually more serious. Complete obstruction in any part of the small or large bowel, if untreated, can cause death within hours due to shock and vascular collapse. Intestinal obstruction is most likely to occur after abdominal surgery or in persons with congenital bowel deformities.

Obstruction in the small intestine results in metabolic alkalosis from dehydration and loss of gastric hydrochloric acid; lower-bowel obstruction causes slower dehydration and loss of intestinal alkaline fluids, resulting in metabolic acidosis. Ultimately, intestinal obstruction may lead to ischemia, necrosis, and death.

Intestinal obstruction develops in three forms.

Simple— Blockage prevents intestinal contents from passing, with no other complications.	*Strangulated—* In addition to blockage of the lumen, blood supply to part or all of the obstructed section is cut off.	*Close-looped—* Both ends of a bowel section are occluded, isolating it from the rest of the intestine.

How it happens

The physiologic effects are similar in all three forms of obstruction. When intestinal obstruction occurs, fluid, air, and gas collect near the obstruction. Peristalsis increases temporarily as the bowel tries to force its contents through the obstruction, injuring intestinal mucosa and causing distention at and above the site of the obstruction. Distention blocks the flow of venous blood and halts normal absorptive processes; as a result, the bowel wall becomes edematous and begins to secrete water, sodium, and potassium into the fluid pooled in the lumen.

Three causes of intestinal obstruction

1 Intussusception with invagination or shortening of the bowel caused by the involution of one segment of the bowel into another.

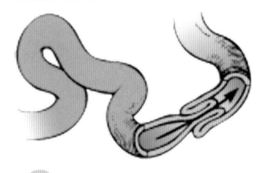

2 Volvulus of the sigmoid colon; the twist is counterclockwise in most cases.

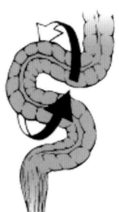

3 Hernia (inguinal); the sac of the hernia is a continuation of the peritoneum of the abdomen. The hernial contents are intestine, omentum, or other abdominal contents that pass through the hernial opening into the hernial sac.

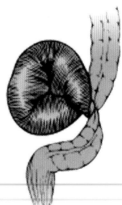

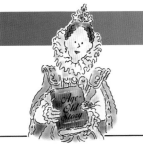

Age-old story

Age and intestinal obstruction

Intussusception, or the telescoping of the bowel into another segment, is the most common cause of intestinal obstruction in children younger than age 2.

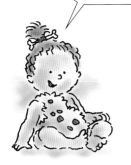

If you suspect I have intestinal obstruction, it's probably intussusception. Boy that's a long word!

What to look for

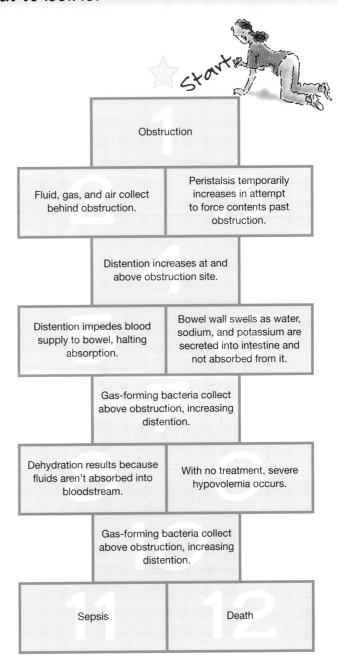

Start

1. Obstruction

2. Fluid, gas, and air collect behind obstruction.

3. Peristalsis temporarily increases in attempt to force contents past obstruction.

4. Distention increases at and above obstruction site.

5. Distention impedes blood supply to bowel, halting absorption.

6. Bowel wall swells as water, sodium, and potassium are secreted into intestine and not absorbed from it.

7. Gas-forming bacteria collect above obstruction, increasing distention.

8. Dehydration results because fluids aren't absorbed into bloodstream.

9. With no treatment, severe hypovolemia occurs.

10. Gas-forming bacteria collect above obstruction, increasing distention.

11. Sepsis

12. Death

Ulcerative colitis

Ulcerative colitis is an inflammatory disease that affects the mucosa of the colon and rectum. It invariably begins in the rectum and sigmoid colon, rarely affecting the small intestine, except for the terminal ileum. Ulcerative colitis produces edema (leading to mucosal friability) and ulcerations. The disease cycles between exacerbation and remission. It damages the large intestine's mucosal and submucosal layers.

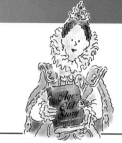

Age-old story

Age and ulcerative colitis

Ulcerative colitis occurs primarily in young adults. Onset of symptoms seems to occur most commonly between ages 15 and 30 and between ages 55 and 65.

How it happens

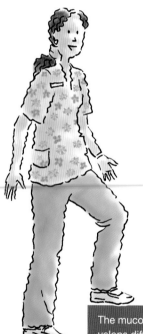

Usually, the disease originates in the rectum and lower colon. Then it spreads to the entire colon.

The mucosa develops diffuse ulceration, with hemorrhage, congestion, edema, and exudative inflammation. Ulcerations are continuous (unlike Crohn's disease).

Abscesses formed in the mucosa drain purulent pus, become necrotic, and ulcerate.

Sloughing occurs, causing bloody, mucus-filled stools.

Ch-ch-changes...I used to have a normal colon attached, but with the progression of ulcerative colitis, my buddy the colon has gone through some changes...

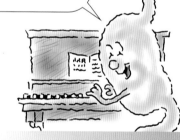

- Initially, the colon's mucosal surface becomes dark, red, and velvety.
- Abscesses form and coalesce into ulcers.
- Necrosis of the mucosa occurs.
- As abscesses heal, scarring and thickening may appear in the bowel's inner muscle layer.
- As granulation tissue replaces the muscle layer, the colon narrows, shortens, and loses its characteristic pouches (haustral folds).

Mucosal changes in ulcerative colitis

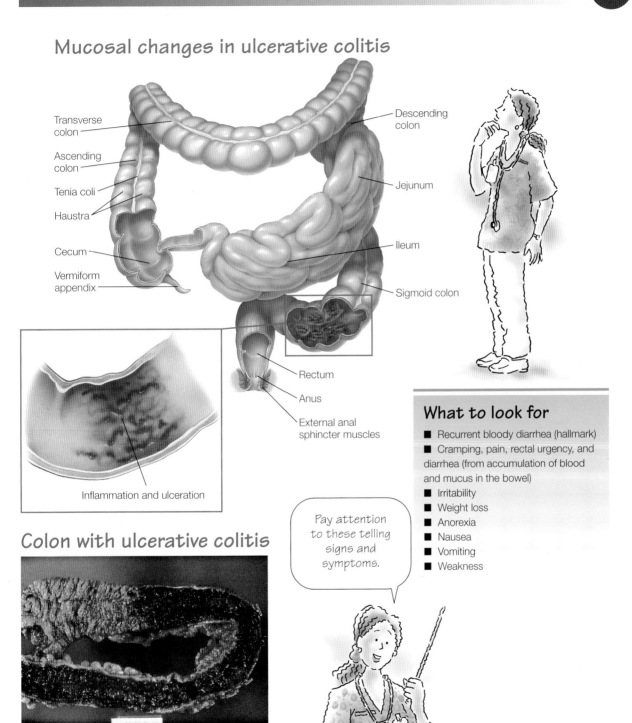

Transverse colon

Ascending colon

Tenia coli

Haustra

Cecum

Vermiform appendix

Descending colon

Jejunum

Ileum

Sigmoid colon

Rectum

Anus

External anal sphincter muscles

Inflammation and ulceration

What to look for

■ Recurrent bloody diarrhea (hallmark)
■ Cramping, pain, rectal urgency, and diarrhea (from accumulation of blood and mucus in the bowel)
■ Irritability
■ Weight loss
■ Anorexia
■ Nausea
■ Vomiting
■ Weakness

Pay attention to these telling signs and symptoms.

Colon with ulcerative colitis

Prominent erythema and ulceration of the colon begin in the ascending colon and are most severe in the rectosigmoid area.

VISION QUEST

Show and tell

Name the two types of diverticular disease shown at right and then define them.

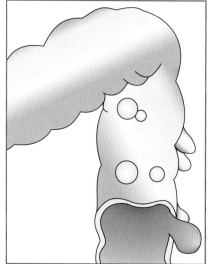 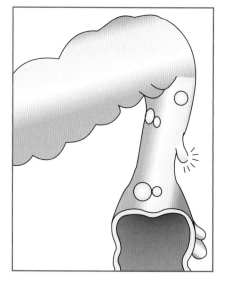

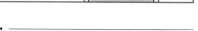
1. _____

2. _____

Rebus riddle

Solve the riddle to find out a way to help avoid many GI disorders, including colorectal cancer.

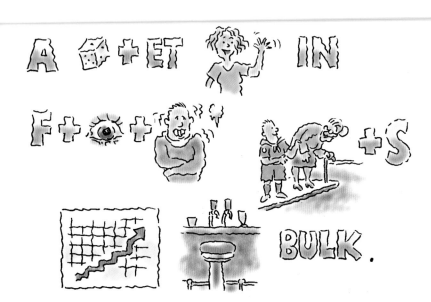

6 Musculoskeletal disorders

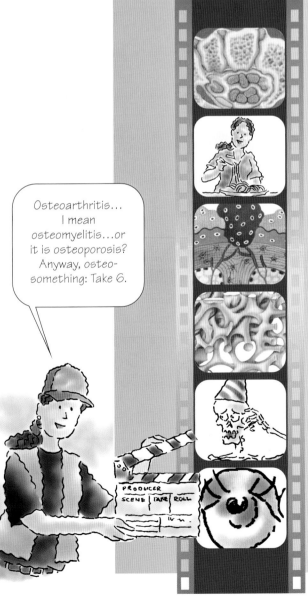

Osteoarthritis... I mean osteomyelitis...or it is osteoporosis? Anyway, osteo-something: Take 6.

Carpal tunnel syndrome

The most common of the nerve entrapment syndromes, carpal tunnel syndrome (CTS) results from compression of the median nerve at the wrist within the carpal tunnel.

Continuous or periodic compression on a nerve can cause damage over time. Certain nerves are located in regions of the body that are especially vulnerable to compression injuries. The carpal tunnel is one such region.

How it happens

The carpal bones and the transverse carpal ligament form the carpal tunnel. Inflammation or fibrosis of the tendon sheaths that pass through the carpal tunnel usually causes edema and compression of the median nerve. This compression neuropathy causes sensory and motor changes in the median distribution of the hands, initially impairing sensory transmission to the thumb, index finger, middle (second) finger, and inner aspect of the ring (fourth) finger.

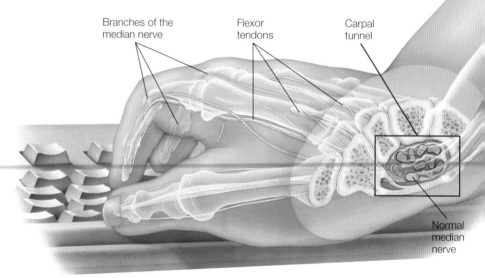

Branches of the median nerve

Flexor tendons

Carpal tunnel

Normal median nerve

Rheumatoid arthritis

Systemic disorders, such as diabetes, rheumatoid arthritis, hypothyroidism, and amyloidosis can be a risk factor.

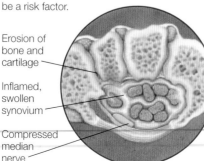

Erosion of bone and cartilage

Inflamed, swollen synovium

Compressed median nerve

Repetitive trauma

Repetitive movements expose the nerve to compression forces and stretching.

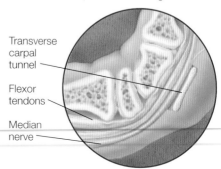

Transverse carpal tunnel

Flexor tendons

Median nerve

Risky business
Risk factors for carpal tunnel

- Female gender
- Age 40 or older
- Job or hobbies that involve highly repetitive tasks
- Diabetes
- Rheumatoid arthritis
- Hypothyroidism
- Pregnancy
- Trauma to wrist
- Menopause
- Obesity

One of the main risk factors for carpal tunnel is a job that requires repetitive tasks.

No bones about it... carpal tunnel syndrome can be very painful.

Cross section of the wrist with CTS

Increased pressure on the median nerve decreases blood flow. If compression persists, the nerve begins to swell. The myelin sheath begins to thin and degenerate.

Carpal bones:
- Hamate
- Capitate
- Trapezoid
- Trapezium

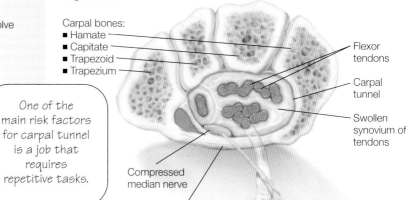
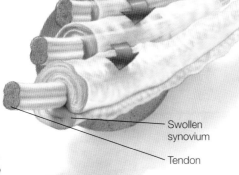

Flexor tendons

Carpal tunnel

Swollen synovium of tendons

Compressed median nerve

Transverse carpal ligament

Flexor tendon in synovium

Nerve fiber

Capillary plexus

Degenerated myelin sheath

Basal lamina

Normal myelin sheath

Axon of nerve

Swollen synovium

Tendon

What to look for

- Weakness, pain, burning, numbness, or tingling in one or both hands
- Paresthesia that affects the thumb, index finger, middle finger, and ring or fourth finger
- Inability to clench the hand into a fist
- Atrophic nails
- Dry and shiny skin

Herniated disk

A herniated disk, also called a *ruptured* or *slipped disk* or *herniated nucleus pulposus*, occurs when all or part of the nucleus pulposus—the soft, gelatinous, central portion of the intervertebral disk—protrudes through the disk's weakened or torn outer ring *(anulus fibrosus)*.

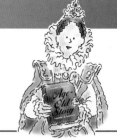

Age-old story

Age and herniated disks

A herniated disk occurs more frequently in middle-aged and older men.

> In older patients whose disks have begun to degenerate, even minor trauma may cause herniation.

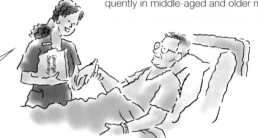

How it happens

An intervertebral disk has two parts: the soft center (nucleus pulposus) and the tough, fibrous surrounding ring (anulus fibrosus). The nucleus pulposus acts as a shock absorber, distributing the mechanical stress applied to the spine when the body moves.

Physical stress, usually a twisting motion, can tear or rupture the anulus fibrosus so that the nucleus pulposus herniates into the spinal canal. The vertebrae move closer together and, in turn, exert pressure on the nerve roots as they exit between the vertebrae. Physical stress, from severe trauma or strain, or intervertebral joint degeneration may cause herniation. Herniation occurs in three stages: protrusion, extrusion, and sequestration.

> Think PESto for your pasta and when you want to remember the three steps in herniation.

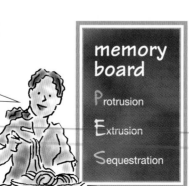

memory board

Protrusion

Extrusion

Sequestration

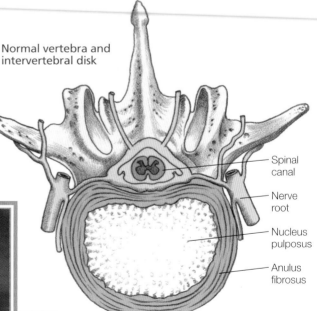

Normal vertebra and intervertebral disk

- Spinal canal
- Nerve root
- Nucleus pulposus
- Anulus fibrosus

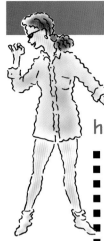

Risky business
Risk factors for herniated disk

- Advancing age
- Male gender
- History of back injury
- Previous herniated disc, or back surgery
- Long periods of sitting, or lifting or pulling heavy objects
- Frequent bending or twisting of the back
- Heavy physical exertion
- Repetitive motions
- Exposure to constant vibration (such as driving)
- Lack of regular exercise
- Strenuous exercise for a long time, or starting to exercise too strenuously after a long period of inactivity
- Smoking
- Being overweight
- Frequent coughing

What to look for

- Severe lower back pain (usually unilateral) to the buttocks, legs, and feet
- Sudden pain after trauma, subsiding after a few days only to return at shorter intervals with progressive intensity
- Sciatic pain after trauma
- Sensory and motor loss in the area innervated by the compressed spinal nerve root
- Weakness and atrophy of leg muscles (later sign)

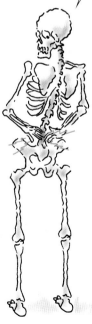

It pains me to say it, but I seem to have a herniated disk!

Protrusion

In protrusion, the nucleus pulposus presses against the anulus fibrosus.

Extrusion and sequestration

In extrusion, the nucleus pulposus bulges forcibly through the anulus fibrosus, pushing against the nerve root. Sequestration occurs when the anulus gives way as the disk's core bursts and presses against the nerve root.

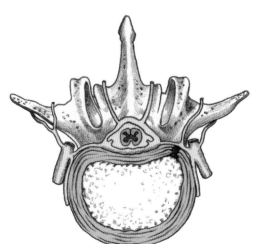

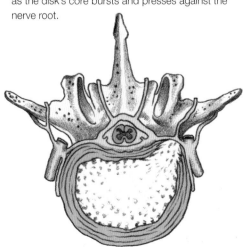

Osteoarthritis

Osteoarthritis, the most common form of arthritis, is widespread, occurring equally in both genders. Symptoms appear after age 40; its earliest symptoms generally begin in middle age and may progress with advancing age.

The rate of progression varies, and joints may remain stable for years in an early stage of deterioration.

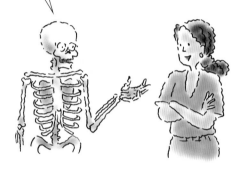

> With osteoarthritis, the degree of disability depends on the site of involvement and its severity. I can have minor finger limitation or severe knee disability.

How it happens

Osteoarthritis is chronic, causing deterioration of the joint cartilage and formation of reactive new bone at the margins and subchondral (below the cartilage) areas of the joints. This degeneration results from a breakdown of chondrocytes (cartilage cells), most commonly in the hips and knees.

Articular cartilage
Death of chondrocytes
Tide mark
Calcified cartilage
Subchondral bone plate
Marrow

1 Chondrocytes break down in the articular cartilage.

Cloning of chondrocytes
Synovial fluid
Deep crack through tide mark with underlying neovascularization
Osteoblast
Osteoclast

3 Cartilage is gradually worn away as a result of the degeneration of the cartilage and leakage of synovial fluid.

Synovial fluid leaks into crack
Early cracking and fibrillation of cartilage

2 The death of chondrocytes forms a crack in the articular cartilage. Synovial fluid leaks out as the cartilage degenerates.

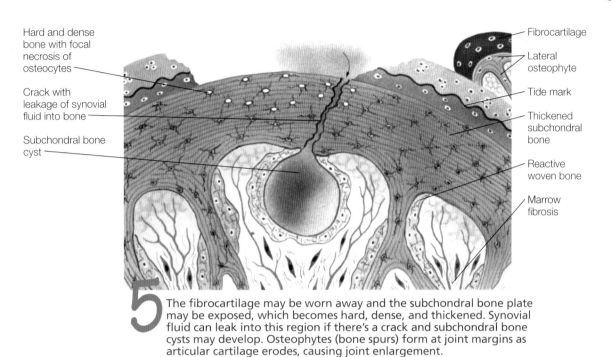

Hard and dense bone with focal necrosis of osteocytes

Crack with leakage of synovial fluid into bone

Subchondral bone cyst

Fibrocartilage

Lateral osteophyte

Tide mark

Thickened subchondral bone

Reactive woven bone

Marrow fibrosis

5 The fibrocartilage may be worn away and the subchondral bone plate may be exposed, which becomes hard, dense, and thickened. Synovial fluid can leak into this region if there's a crack and subchondral bone cysts may develop. Osteophytes (bone spurs) form at joint margins as articular cartilage erodes, causing joint enlargement.

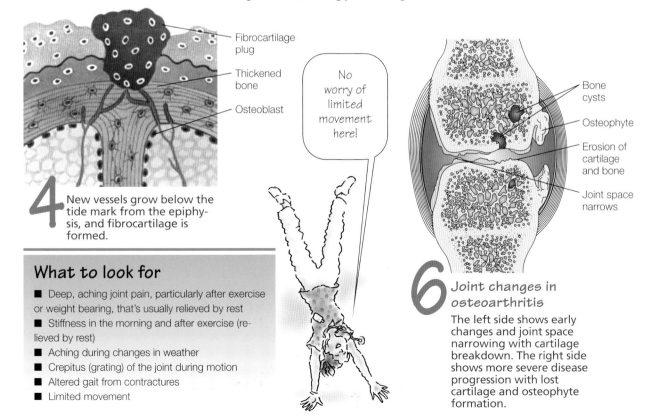

Fibrocartilage plug

Thickened bone

Osteoblast

4 New vessels grow below the tide mark from the epiphysis, and fibrocartilage is formed.

No worry of limited movement here!

What to look for

■ Deep, aching joint pain, particularly after exercise or weight bearing, that's usually relieved by rest
■ Stiffness in the morning and after exercise (relieved by rest)
■ Aching during changes in weather
■ Crepitus (grating) of the joint during motion
■ Altered gait from contractures
■ Limited movement

Bone cysts

Osteophyte

Erosion of cartilage and bone

Joint space narrows

6 Joint changes in osteoarthritis

The left side shows early changes and joint space narrowing with cartilage breakdown. The right side shows more severe disease progression with lost cartilage and osteophyte formation.

Osteomyelitis

Osteomyelitis is a bone infection characterized by progressive inflammatory destruction after formation of new bone. It commonly results from a combination of local trauma—usually trivial but causing a hematoma—and an acute infection originating elsewhere in the body. It may be chronic or acute.

Chronic osteomyelitis, which is rare, is characterized by draining sinus tracts and widespread lesions.

Acute osteomyelitis is usually a blood-borne disease and most commonly affects rapidly growing children.

How it happens

Typically, organisms find a culture site in a hematoma (from recent trauma) or in a weakened area, such as the site of local infection (for example, furunculosis), and travel through the bloodstream to the metaphysis, the section of a long bone that's continuous with the epiphysis plates, where the blood flows into sinusoids.

The most common pyogenic organism in osteomyelitis is *Staphylococcus aureus*.

Stages of osteomyelitis

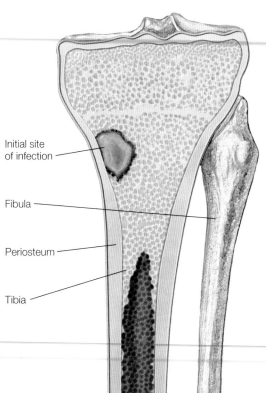

Initial infection

Initial site of infection

Fibula

Periosteum

Tibia

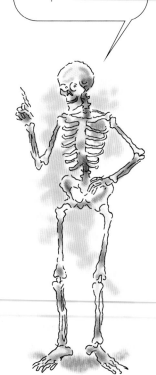

Although osteomyelitis typically remains localized, it can spread through the bone to the marrow, cortex, and periosteum.

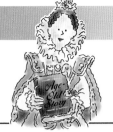

What to look for

■ Rapid onset with sudden pain in the affected bone
■ Tenderness
■ Heat
■ Swelling
■ Erythema
■ Guarding of the affected region of the limb
■ Restricted movement
■ Chronic infection presenting intermittently for years, flaring after minor trauma or persisting as drainage of pus from an old pocket in a sinus tract
■ Fever
■ Dehydration (in children)
■ Irritability and poor feeding in infants

Age-old story

Age and osteomyelitis

Osteomyelitis is more common in children (especially boys) than in adults—usually as a complication of an acute localized infection. Typical sites in children are the lower end of the femur and the upper ends of the tibia, humerus, and radius. The most common sites in adults are the pelvis and vertebrae, generally after surgery or trauma.

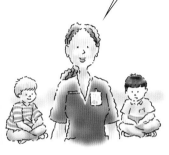

Osteomyelitis is more common in children, especially boys.

First stage

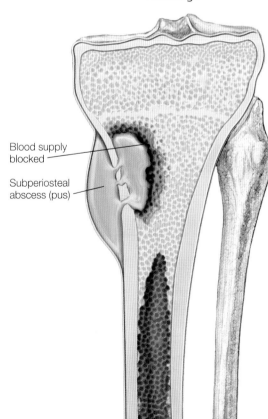

Blood supply blocked

Subperiosteal abscess (pus)

Second stage

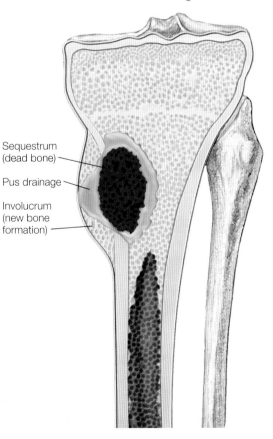

Sequestrum (dead bone)

Pus drainage

Involucrum (new bone formation)

Osteoporosis

Osteoporosis is a metabolic bone disorder in which the rate of bone resorption accelerates and the rate of bone formation decelerates. The result is decreased bone mass. Bones affected by this disease lose calcium and phosphate and become porous, brittle, and abnormally prone to fracture.

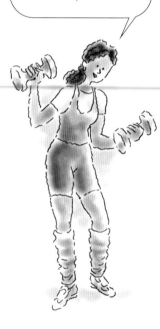

> It's best to build those muscles and strengthen those bones to avoid osteoporosis.

How it happens

In normal bone, the rates of bone formation and resorption are constant; replacement follows resorption immediately, and the amount of bone replaced equals the amount of bone resorbed. Blood absorbs calcium (Ca^{++}) from the digestive system and deposits it in the bones.

Osteoporosis develops when the remodeling cycle is interrupted and new bone formation falls behind resorption. When bone is resorbed faster than it forms, the bone becomes less dense. Men have about 30% greater bone mass than women, which may explain why osteoporosis occurs most often in women and develops later in men.

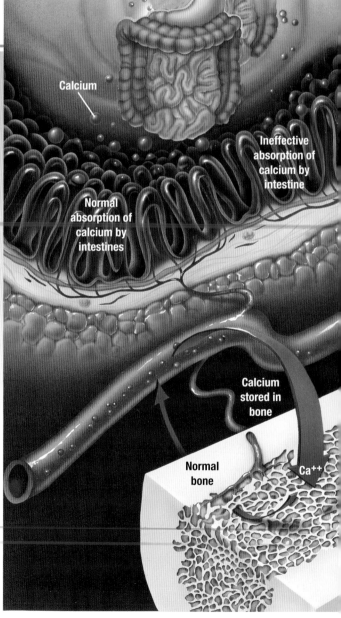

Calcium

Ineffective absorption of calcium by intestine

Normal absorption of calcium by intestines

Calcium stored in bone

Normal bone

Ca^{++}

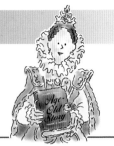

Age and osteoporosis

Primary osteoporosis is often called *senile* or *post-menopausal* osteoporosis because it most commonly develops in postmenopausal women; estogen supports normal bone metabolism.

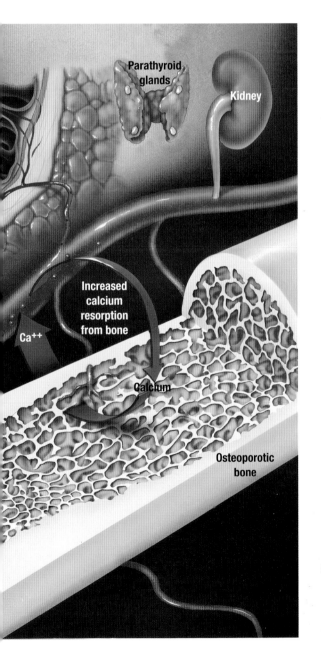

Parathyroid glands

Kidney

Increased calcium resorption from bone

Ca++

Calcium

Osteoporotic bone

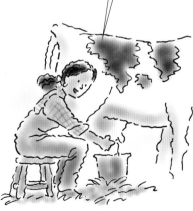

Calcium is key to building and maintaining bone mass. Right, Bessie?

What to look for

- Loss of height
- Spinal deformity (kyphosis)
- Spontaneous wedge fractures
- Pathologic fractures of the neck and femur
- Colles' fractures
- Vertebral collapse
- Hip fractures
- Pain

Bone formation and reabsorption

The organic portion of bone, called *osteoid,* acts as the matrix or framework for the mineral portion. Bone cells, called *osteoblasts,* produce the osteoid matrix. The mineral portion, which consists of calcium and other minerals, hardens the osteoid matrix.

Large bone cells, called *osteoblasts,* reshape mature bones by resorbing the mineral and organic components. However, in osteoporosis, osteoblasts continue to produce bone, but resorption by osteoclasts exceeds bone formation.

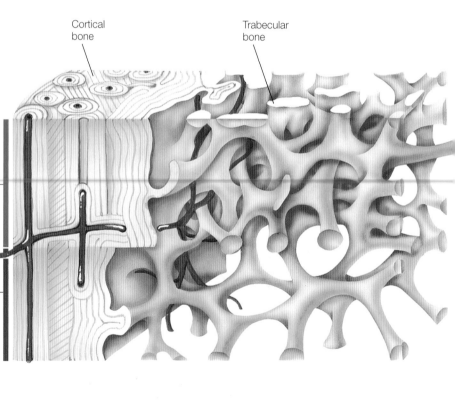

I could have sworn I was taller last year.

Normal bone

Osteoporotic bone

Cortical bone

Trabecular bone

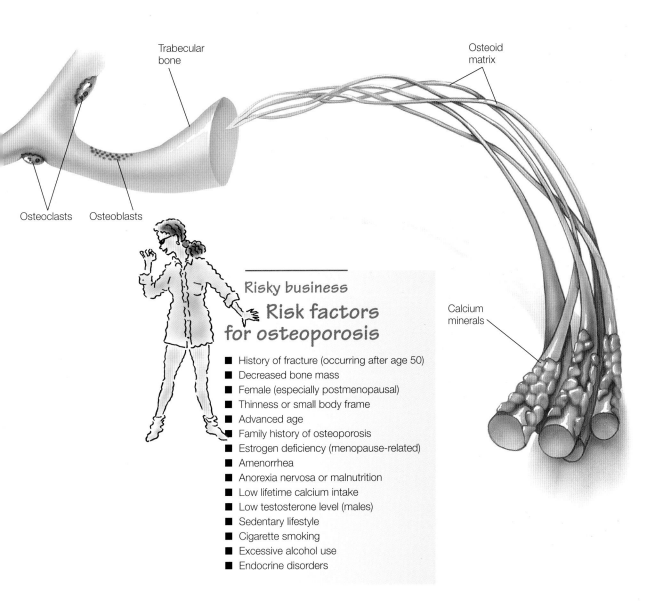

Trabecular bone

Osteoid matrix

Osteoclasts   Osteoblasts

Calcium minerals

Risky business
Risk factors for osteoporosis

- History of fracture (occurring after age 50)
- Decreased bone mass
- Female (especially postmenopausal)
- Thinness or small body frame
- Advanced age
- Family history of osteoporosis
- Estrogen deficiency (menopause-related)
- Amenorrhea
- Anorexia nervosa or malnutrition
- Low lifetime calcium intake
- Low testosterone level (males)
- Sedentary lifestyle
- Cigarette smoking
- Excessive alcohol use
- Endocrine disorders

Osteosarcoma

Osteosarcoma is a highly aggressive malignant bone tumor usually occurring during periods of bone growth. It most commonly occurs in the extremities of long bones near metaphyseal growth plates. Although it can occur in any bone, it tends to appear most frequently in bones that have the fastest bone growth, such as the lower femur or upper tibia or fibula. The humerus is the second most common site.

How it happens

Osteosarcomas are growths of abnormal cells in bones. These abnormal cells divide uncontrollably and healthy tissue is replaced with un-healthy tissue. Osteosarcomas grow rapidly and move from the metaphysis of the bone to the periosteal surface.

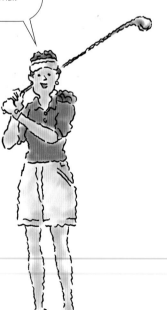

All *humerus* aside...the lower femur, upper tibia and fibula (and humerus) are the *fore* sites most often affected by osteosarcoma.

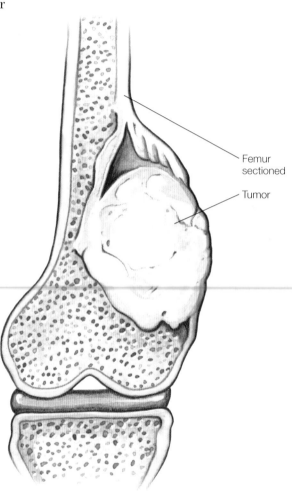

Femur sectioned

Tumor

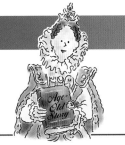

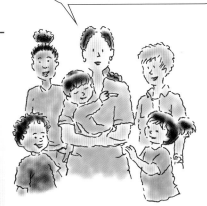

Osteosarcoma is the most common bone tumor in children and the third most common bone cancer in children and adolescents.

Age-old story

Age and osteosarcoma

Osteosarcoma tumors occur equally in male and female adolescents. In females, they usually occur by age 15; in males, after age 15.

Osteosarcoma in the distal femur

In the distal femur, osteosarcoma has extended through the cortex of the bone into the soft tissue and the bony epiphysis.

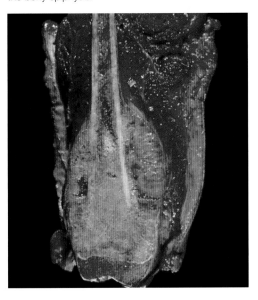

What to look for

- Deep, localized pain
- Nighttime awakening with pain
- Swelling in the affected bone
- Sudden onset of pain
- Shiny skin over tumor that's stretched with prominent superficial veins

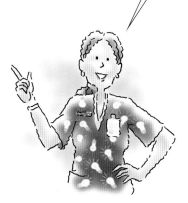

These are the five things to look for when checking for signs and symptoms of osteosarcomas.

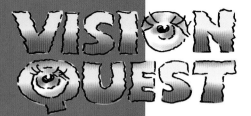

VISION QUEST

Able to label?

In this illustration, label the parts of the hand involved in carpal tunnel syndrome.

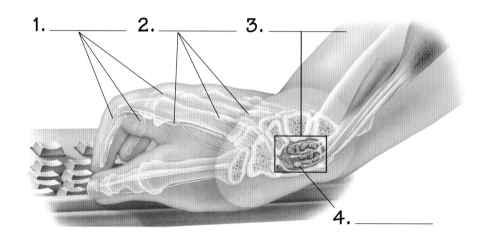

1. _____
2. _____
3. _____
4. _____

My word!

Solve the word scrambles to identify parts of the musculoskeletal system. Then rearrange the circled letters to answer the question posed.

Question: What's the most common form of arthritis in adults?

1. gecailart ＿＿＿＿◯◯＿＿＿◯
2. tjnsoi ＿◯＿＿◯＿
3. regsnif ＿◯＿＿＿◯
4. nseke ＿＿＿＿◯
5. onbcsuladrh ＿＿＿＿＿◯＿＿＿◯◯＿
6. drchyoncoest ＿＿◯＿＿＿＿＿＿◯＿◯

Answer: ＿＿＿＿＿＿＿＿＿＿＿＿＿＿

7 Hematologic disorders

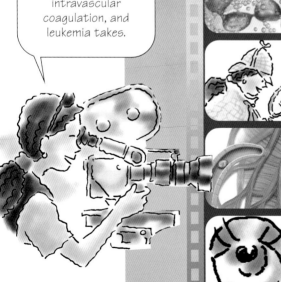

OK, sickle cells, you're in my scene. Please move out of the camera until we finish with the anemia, disseminated intravascular coagulation, and leukemia takes.

Anemia, folic acid deficiency

Folic acid deficiency anemia is a common, slowly progressive, megaloblastic anemia.

How it happens

Folic acid (pteroylglutamic acid, folacin) is found in most body tissues, where it acts as a coenzyme in metabolic processes involving one-carbon transfer. It's essential for the formation and maturation of red blood cells (RBCs) and the synthesis of deoxyribonucleic acid. Although its body stores are relatively small (about 70 mg), this vitamin is plentiful in most well-balanced diets.

Even so, because folic acid is water-soluble and heat-labile, it's easily destroyed in the cooking process. Also, about 20% of folic acid taken in through diet is excreted unabsorbed. Insufficient daily folic acid intake (less than 50 mcg/day) usually induces folic acid deficiency within 4 months, as the body stores in the liver are depleted.

This deficiency inhibits cell growth, particularly RBCs, leading to production of few, deformed RBCs. These enlarged red cells characteristic of the megaloblastic anemias have a shortened life span—weeks rather than months.

The lowdown on low folic acid

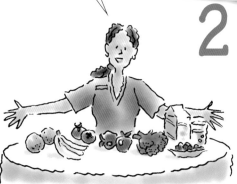

Get the point? I need my folic acid.

A well-balanced diet provides a healthy supply of folic acid.

2 Depleted body stores in liver

1 Insufficient folic acid intake (less than 50 mcg/day) or malabsorption

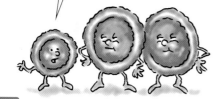

I wish I were big!

3 Inhibition of RBC growth

Gasp! I don't want a shortened life span!

4 Production of few, deformed RBCs with shortened life spans

What to look for

- Anorexia
- Fainting
- Weakness
- Progressive fatigue
- Shortness of breath
- Palpitations
- Forgetfulness
- Glossitis
- Headache
- Irritability
- Nausea
- Pallor

Why, you're even smaller than the nucleus of a lymphocyte!

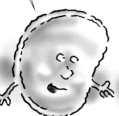
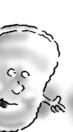

5 RBCs smaller than the nucleus of a lymphocyte

Take A SWING at some signs and symptoms of folic acid deficiency.

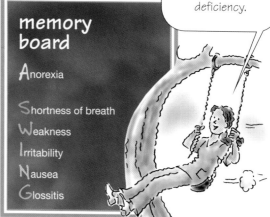

memory board

Anorexia

Shortness of breath

Weakness

Irritability

Nausea

Glossitis

Anemia, iron deficiency

Iron deficiency anemia is a disorder of oxygen transport in which hemoglobin synthesis is deficient. A common disease worldwide, iron deficiency anemia affects 10% to 30% of the adult population of the United States. The prognosis after replacement therapy is favorable.

How it happens

Iron deficiency anemia occurs when the supply of iron is too low for optimal RBC formation. The low iron supply results in smaller (microcytic) cells that contain less color when they're stained for visualization under a microscope.

When the body uses up its iron stores, including plasma iron, the concentration of transferrin, which binds with and transports iron, decreases. Insufficient iron stores lead to smaller than normal RBCs that have a lower than normal hemoglobin concentration. In turn, the blood carries less oxygen.

I knew I should have taken my iron today.

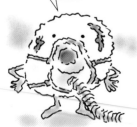

Peripheral blood smear in iron deficiency anemia

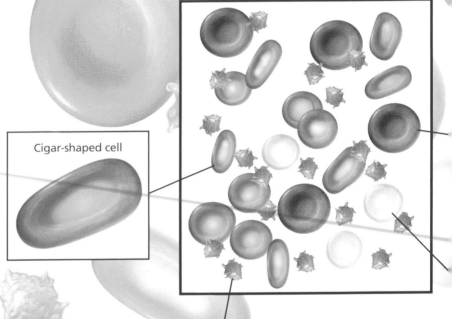

Cigar-shaped cell

Platelet

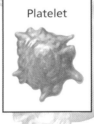

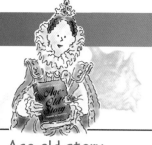

Age-old story

Age and iron deficiency anemia

Iron deficiency anemia is most common in premenopausal women, infants (particularly premature or low-birth-weight infants), children, and adolescents (especially girls).

Risky business

Risk factors for iron deficiency anemia

Insufficient intake

- Vegetarian diet
- Macrobiotic diet
- Low intake of meat, fish, poultry, or iron-fortified foods (including conditions resulting in malabsorption)
- Low intake of foods rich in ascorbic acid
- Frequent dieting or restricted eating
- Chronic or significant weight loss
- Substance abuse

Excessive use

- Heavy or lengthy menstrual periods
- Rapid growth
- Pregnancy (recent or current)
- Inflammatory bowel disease
- Chronic use of aspirin or nonsteroidal anti-inflammatory drugs such as ibuprofen
- Corticosteroid use
- Participation in endurance sports (long-distance running, swimming, cycling)
- Intensive physical training
- Frequent blood donations
- Parasitic infection

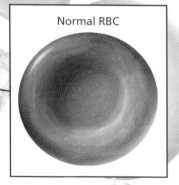

Normal RBC

Microcytic, hypochromic RBC

What to look for

- Exertional dyspnea, fatigue, listlessness, pallor, inability to concentrate, irritability, headache, and susceptibility to infection
- Increased cardiac output and tachycardia
- Coarsely ridged, spoon-shaped (koilonychia), brittle, thin nails
- Sore, red, burning tongue
- Sore, dry skin in the corners of the mouth
- Blue tinge to sclerae

Anemia, pernicious

Pernicious anemia, the most common type of megaloblastic anemia, is caused by malabsorption of vitamin B_{12}. It's characterized by a lack of intrinsic factor, which is needed to absorb vitamin B_{12}, and widespread RBC destruction.

   If not treated, pernicious anemia is fatal. Its manifestations subside with treatment, but some neurologic deficits caused by this condition may be permanent.

How it happens

Pernicious anemia is characterized by decreased production of hydrochloric acid in the stomach and a deficiency of intrinsic factor, which is normally secreted by the parietal cells of the gastric mucosa and is essential for vitamin B_{12} absorption in the ileum. The resulting vitamin B_{12} deficiency inhibits cell growth, particularly of RBCs, leading to production of few, deformed RBCs with poor oxygen-carrying capacity. It also causes neurologic damage by impairing myelin formation.

Peripheral blood smear in pernicious anemia

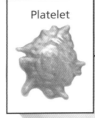

Platelet

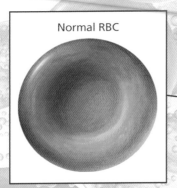

Normal RBC

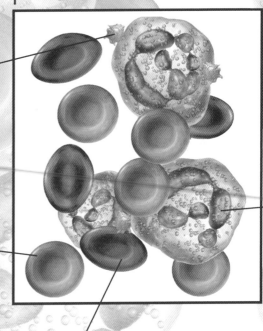

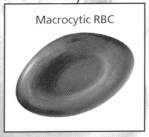

Macrocytic RBC

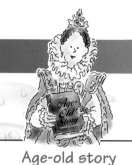

Age and pernicious anemia

The onset of pernicious anemia typically occurs between ages 50 and 60, and incidence increases with age. Elderly patients commonly have a dietary deficiency of vitamin B_{12} in addition to or instead of poor absorption.

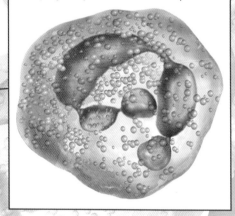

Hypersegmented polymorphonuclear neutrophil

What to look for

> I'd feel much better with a little help from my friend hydrochloric acid.

GI

- Nausea, vomiting, anorexia, weight loss, flatulence, diarrhea, and constipation from disturbed digestion
- Gingival bleeding and tongue inflammation (may hinder eating and intensify anorexia)

> It all started when my myelin broke down.

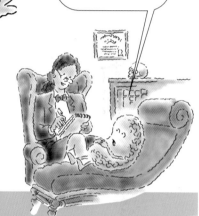

Neurologic

- Neuritis and weakness in the extremities
- Peripheral numbness and paresthesia
- Disturbed position sense
- Lack of coordination, ataxia, and impaired fine finger movement
- Positive Babinski's and Romberg's signs
- Light-headedness
- Altered vision (diplopia, blurred vision), taste, smell, and hearing (tinnitus) and optic muscle atrophy
- Loss of bowel and bladder control
- Impotence (in males) due to demyelination
- Irritability, poor memory, headache, depression, and delirium

> Hey! I shouldn't be doing all the work. Where are those RBCs?

Cardiovascular

- Low hemoglobin level
- Palpitations, wide pulse pressure, dyspnea, orthopnea, tachycardia, premature beats and, eventually, heart failure

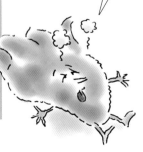

Disseminated intravascular coagulation

> Early detection is crucial! Prognosis depends on it as well as the severity of the hemorrhage and the treatment of the underlying disease.

Disseminated intravascular coagulation (DIC), also called *consumption coagulopathy* or *defibrination syndrome*, is a complication of a disease or condition that accelerates clotting throughout the body. This accelerated clotting causes small blood vessel occlusion, organ necrosis, depletion of circulating clotting factors and platelets, activation of the fibrinolytic system, and consequent severe hemorrhage.

Clotting in the microcirculation (small blood vessels) usually affects the kidneys and extremities, but may occur in the brain, lungs, pituitary and adrenal glands, and GI mucosa. DIC is generally an acute condition but may be chronic in cancer patients.

How it happens

It isn't clear how or why certain disorders lead to DIC. In many patients, the triggering mechanisms may be the entrance of foreign protein into the circulation and vascular endothelial injury.

Regardless of how DIC begins, the typical accelerated clotting results in generalized activation of prothrombin and a consequent excess of thrombin.

Tissue damage in DIC

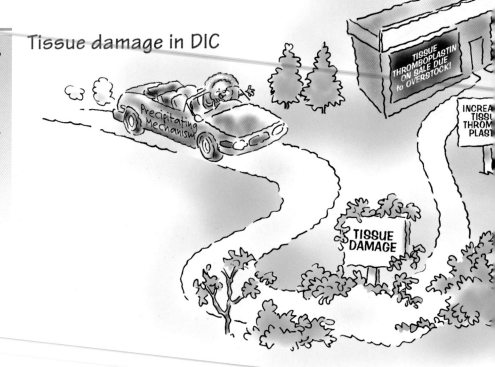

Precipitating Mechanism

TISSUE THROMBOPLASTIN ON SALE DUE to OVERSTOCK!

INCREA TISSU THROM PLAST

TISSUE DAMAGE

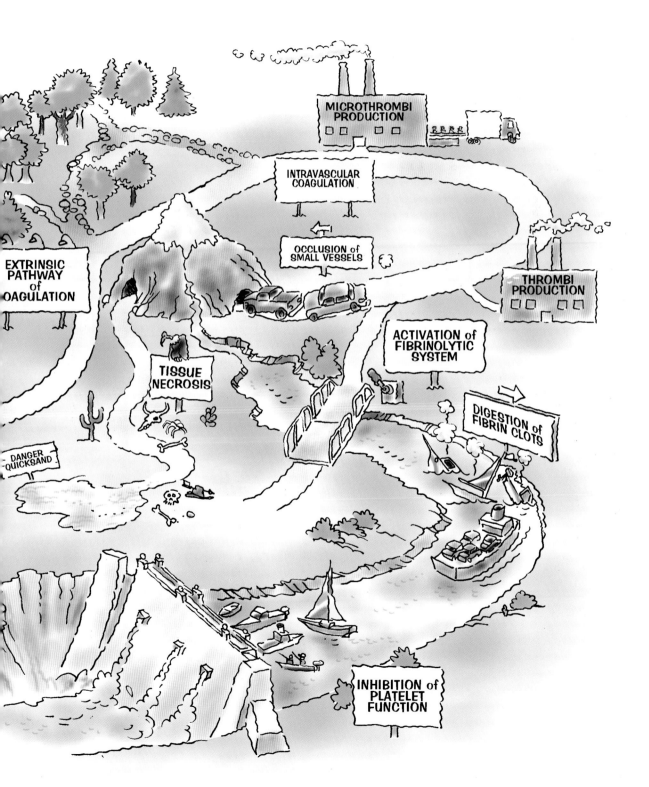

Risky business

Risk factors for DIC

- Infection
- Obstetric complications
- Neoplastic disease
- Disorders that produce necrosis, such as extensive burns and trauma
- Heatstroke
- Shock
- Incompatible blood transfusions
- Drug reactions
- Cardiac arrest
- Surgery necessitating cardiopulmonary bypass
- Acute respiratory distress syndrome
- Diabetic ketoacidosis
- Pulmonary embolism
- Severe liver disease
- Severe head injury

Endothelial damage in DIC

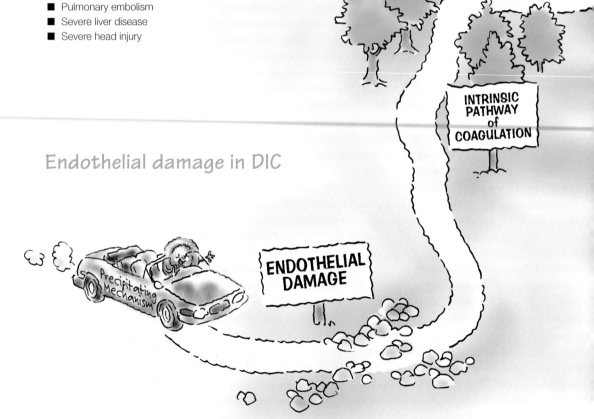

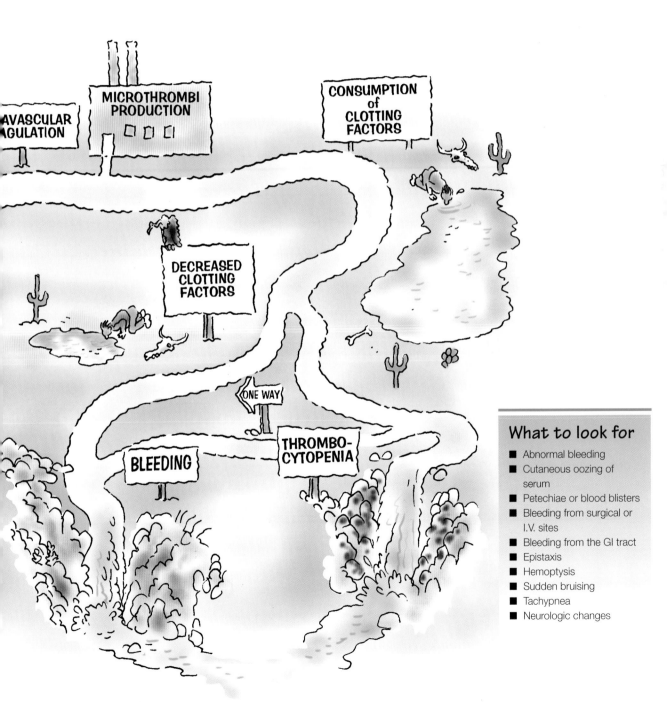

What to look for

- Abnormal bleeding
- Cutaneous oozing of serum
- Petechiae or blood blisters
- Bleeding from surgical or I.V. sites
- Bleeding from the GI tract
- Epistaxis
- Hemoptysis
- Sudden bruising
- Tachypnea
- Neurologic changes

Leukemia

Leukemia refers to a group of malignant disorders characterized by abnormal proliferation and maturation of lymphocytes and nonlymphocytic cells, leading to the suppression of normal cells. It can be classified as *acute* or *chronic*, with subclassifications of *lymphocytic* or *myelogenous*.

How it happens

In leukemia, hematopoietic cells (immature blood cells) undergo an abnormal transformation, giving rise to leukemic cells. Leukemic cells multiply and accumulate, crowding out other types of cells. Crowding prevents production of normal red and white blood cells and platelets, leading to pancytopenia (reduced number of all cellular elements of the blood).

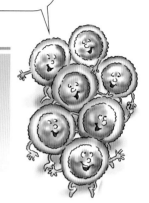

When leukemic cells crowd up, it tends to mean trouble. We get shoved out and pancytopenia results.

Acute lymphocytic leukemia

Abnormal growth of lymphocytic precursors (lymphoblasts)

Acute myelogenous leukemia

Rapid accumulation of myeloid precursors (myeloblasts)

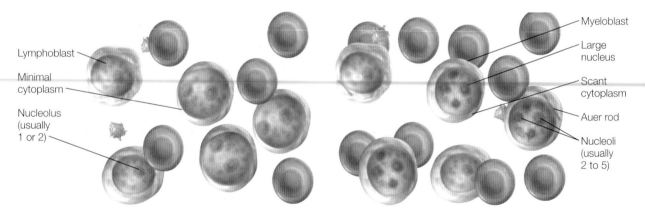

Lymphoblast

Minimal cytoplasm

Nucleolus (usually 1 or 2)

Myeloblast

Large nucleus

Scant cytoplasm

Auer rod

Nucleoli (usually 2 to 5)

What to look for

Acute (lymphocytic and myeloid)

Related to suppression of elements of the bone marrow

- Anemia
- Bleeding
- Fever
- Infection
- Night sweats
- Weight loss
- Paleness
- Lethargy
- Malaise

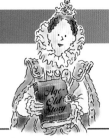

Age and leukemia

Acute lymphocytic leukemia accounts for 80% of childhood cases of leukemia. Treatment leads to remission in 81% of children, who survive an average of 5 years, and in 65% of adults, who survive an average of 2 years. Children ages 2 to 8 who receive intensive therapy have the best survival rate.

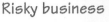

Risk factors for leukemia

- Cigarette smoking
- Exposure to certain chemicals (such as benzene, which is present in cigarette smoke and gasoline)
- Exposure to large doses of ionizing radiation or drugs that depress the bone marrow

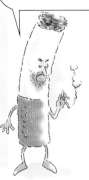

Smoking, along with exposure to certain chemicals, drugs, or ionizing radiation, can cause leukemia.

Chronic lymphocytic leukemia

Uncontrollable spread of small, abnormal lymphocytes in lymphoid tissue, blood, and bone marrow

Chronic myelogenous leukemia

Abnormal overgrowth of granulocytic precursors (myeloblasts, promyelocytes, metamyelocytes, and myelocytes) in bone marrow, blood, and body tissue

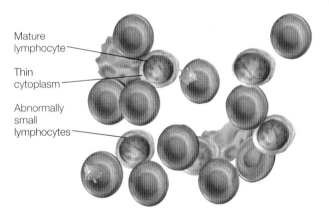

Mature lymphocyte

Thin cytoplasm

Abnormally small lymphocytes

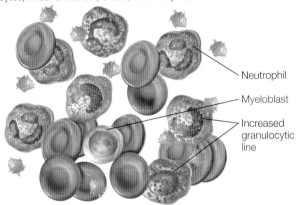

Neutrophil

Myeloblast

Increased granulocytic line

Chronic lymphocytic

Early
- Fatigue
- Malaise
- Fever
- Nodular enlargement

Late
- Bone tenderness
- Liver or spleen enlargement
- Severe fatigue
- Weight loss

Chronic myelogenous
- Anemia
- Thrombocytopenia
- Ankle edema
- Anorexia, weight loss
- Hepatosplenomegaly
- Prolonged infection
- Low-grade fever
- Renal calculi or gouty arthritis
- Sternal and rib tenderness
- Increased sweating

Sickle cell disease

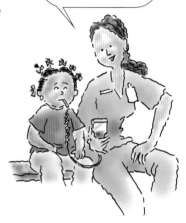

Race has a lot to do with susceptibility to sickle cell disease.

Sickle cell disease is a congenital hemolytic anemia resulting from defective hemoglobin molecules. In the past, patients with sickle cell disease died in their early 20s, and few lived to middle age. Today, however, the average life expectancy is age 45, with 40% to 50% of patients living into their 50s.

Sickle cell disease occurs primarily in persons of African and Mediterranean descent, but it also affects other populations, such as those indigenous to Puerto Rico, Turkey, India, and the Middle East. About 1 in 10 blacks carry the abnormal gene, and 1 in every 400 to 600 black children has sickle cell disease.

How it happens

Sickle cell disease results from the substitution of the amino acid valine for glutamic acid in the hemoglobin S gene, which is an abnormality found in the RBCs of patients with sickle cell disease and which becomes insoluble during hypoxia. As a result, these blood cells become rigid, rough, and elongated, forming a sickle (crescent) shape, which causes hemolysis (disintegration of the cell and release of hemoglobin). The altered cells also pile up in the capillaries and smaller blood vessels, making the blood more viscous. Normal circulation is impaired, causing pain, tissue infarctions, and swelling.

Each patient with sickle cell disease has a different hypoxic threshold and different factors that trigger a sickle cell crisis, in which the sickled blood cells block small blood vessels. Illness, exposure to cold, stress, acidosis, or dehydration precipitates a crisis in most patients. The blood vessel blockages then cause anoxic changes that lead to further sickling and obstruction.

Blood smear in sickle cell disease

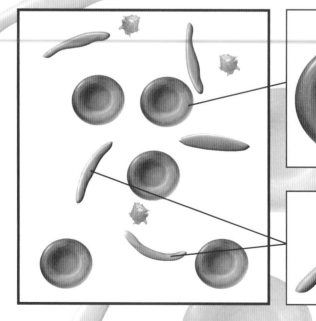

Normal RBC

Sickled cells

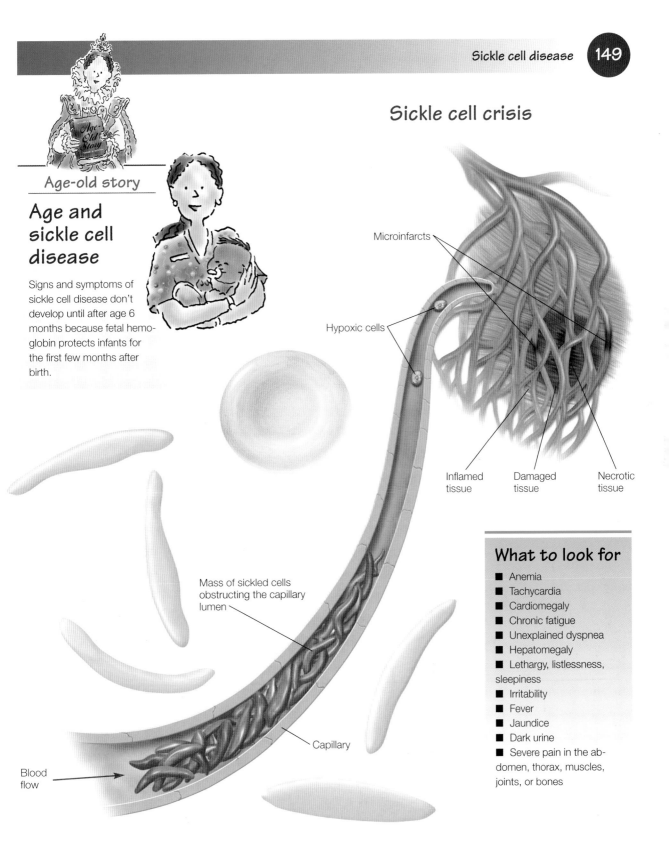

Sickle cell crisis

Microinfarcts

Hypoxic cells

Inflamed tissue

Damaged tissue

Necrotic tissue

Age-old story

Age and sickle cell disease

Signs and symptoms of sickle cell disease don't develop until after age 6 months because fetal hemoglobin protects infants for the first few months after birth.

Mass of sickled cells obstructing the capillary lumen

Capillary

Blood flow

What to look for

- Anemia
- Tachycardia
- Cardiomegaly
- Chronic fatigue
- Unexplained dyspnea
- Hepatomegaly
- Lethargy, listlessness, sleepiness
- Irritability
- Fever
- Jaundice
- Dark urine
- Severe pain in the abdomen, thorax, muscles, joints, or bones

VISION QUEST

Show and tell

Identify the four types of leukemia shown in these illustrations and differentiate among them.

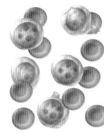 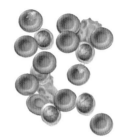 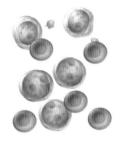 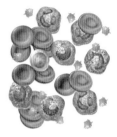

1. _____

2. _____

3. _____

4. _____

Matchmaker

Match the definitions in column 1 with the disorder terms in column 2.

1. Disorder of oxygen transport in which hemoglobin synthesis is deficient ____

2. Common, slowly progressive, megaloblastic leukemia ____

3. Congenital hemolytic anemia resulting from defective hemoglobin molecules ____

4. Complication of a disease or condition that accelerates clotting ____

5. Most common type of megaloblastic anemia; caused by malabsorption of vitamin B_{12} ____

6. Group of malignant disorders characterized by abnormal proliferation and maturation of lymphocytes and nonlymphocytic cells ____

A. Folic acid deficiency anemia

B. Iron deficiency anemia

C. Pernicious anemia

D. DIC

E. Leukemia

F. Sickle cell disease

8
Immune disorders

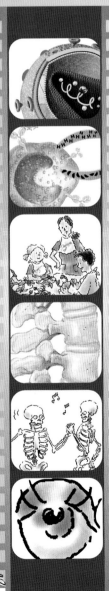

> I'm not *immune* to a little hay fever every once in a while—especially when I'm on location in the South! I feel a sneeze coming on...

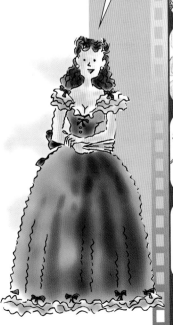

Acquired immunodeficiency syndrome

Acquired immunodeficiency syndrome (AIDS) is thought to be caused by human immunodeficiency virus (HIV) infection. AIDS is characterized by gradual destruction of cell-mediated (T-cell) immunity. However, because AIDS targets the CD4 cells that play a central role in immune reactions, AIDS also affects the other types of immunity:

Humoral immunity:

when foreign substances invade the body; also called an *antibody-mediated response*

Autoimmunity:

when immune cells mistake the body's own cells as invaders and attack them.

The resulting deficiency in immunity makes the patient susceptible to opportunistic infections, cancers, and other abnormalities that characterize AIDS.

How it happens

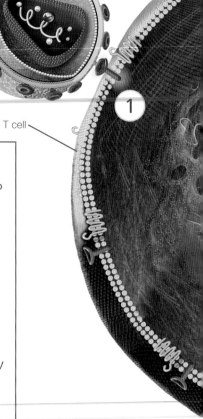

HIV virion

T cell

HIV life cycle

1 HIV binds to the T cell.

2 Viral ribonucleic acid (RNA) is released into the host cell.

3 The viral RNA is converted into viral deoxyribonucleic acid (DNA) through a process called *reverse transcriptase*. During reverse transcriptase, an enzyme reads the sequence of viral RNA nucleic acids that have entered the host cell and transcribes the sequence into a complementary DNA sequence.

4 Viral DNA enters the T cell's nucleus and inserts itself into the T cell's DNA.

5 The T cell begins to make copies of the HIV components.

6 Protease (an enzyme) helps create new virus particles.

7 The new HIV virion (virus particle) is released from the T cell.

Viral RNA

Reverse transcriptase

Viral DNA

Viral RNA

2

3

4   5   6

HIV proteins

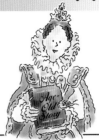

AIDS and children

In children, HIV infection has a mean incubation time of 17 months. Signs and symptoms resemble those seen in adults, except for findings related to sexually transmitted diseases.

Children have a high incidence of opportunistic bacterial infections, such as otitis media, sepsis, chronic salivary gland enlargement, *Mycobacterium avium-intracellulare* complex function, and pneumonias, including lymphoid interstitial pneumonia and *Pneumocystis carinii* pneumonia.

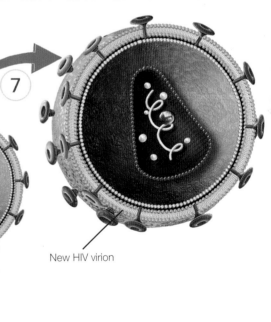

7

New HIV virion

Stages of HIV infection

1. Acute stage

The acute or primary stage of HIV occurs about 1 to 2 weeks after initial infection. During this stage, the virus undergoes massive replication. The patient may be asymptomatic or have flulike symptoms.

2. Asymptomatic HIV

During the asymptomatic stage, chronic signs and symptoms aren't present. T-cell count may be used to monitor progression of the disease. With the patient's own resistance and drug therapy, this stage can last for 10 to 12 years or longer.

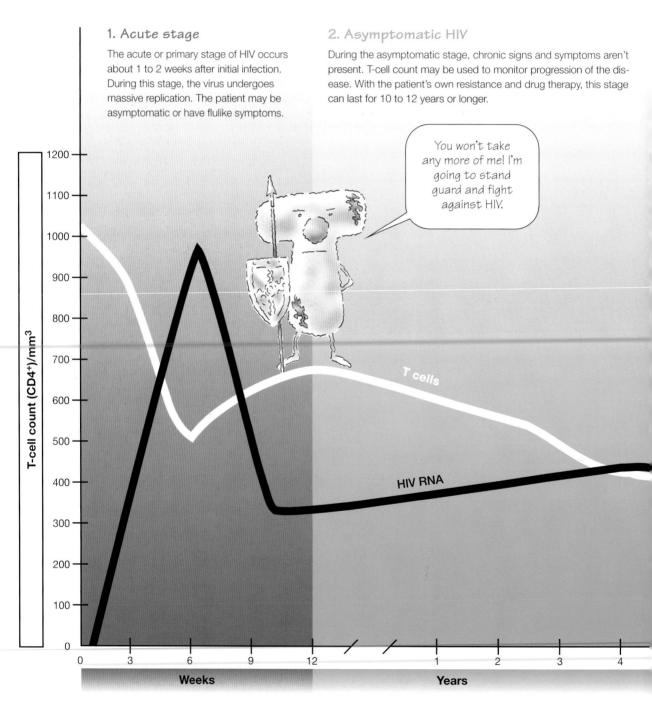

You won't take any more of me! I'm going to stand guard and fight against HIV.

T cells

HIV RNA

T-cell count (CD4+)/mm³

1200
1100
1000
900
800
700
600
500
400
300
200
100
0

0   3   6   9   12   1   2   3   4

Weeks   **Years**

3. Symptomatic HIV

The symptomatic stage has two phases: early and late. When the T-cell count in blood falls below 200 cells/mm^3, it's the late phase. This stage of HIV infection is defined mainly by the emergence of opportunistic infections and cancers to which the immune system normally helps maintain resistance.

4. Advanced HIV

A T-cell count of 50 cells/mm^3 or less represents advanced HIV. With the onset of this phase, patients are at the highest risk for opportunistic infections and malignancies.

What to look for

- Short-term memory loss
- Persistent headaches
- High fever
- Confusion and forgetfulness
- Seizures and lack of co-ordination
- Persistent or frequent oral infections
- Difficulty or pain with swallowing
- Loss of appetite
- Cough and shortness of breath
- Swollen lymph nodes in the neck, armpits, and groin
- Persistent rashes or flaky skin
- Severe weight loss
- Chronic diarrhea
- Lack of energy and muscle weakness

HIV RNA copies per ml plasma

10^7

10^6

10^5

10^4

10^3

10^2

6   7   8   9   10   11

Allergic rhinitis

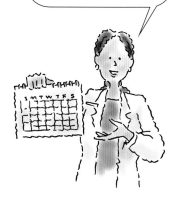

Allergic rhinitis can occur seasonally, such as with hay fever, or year-round, such as with perennial allergic rhinitis.

Allergic rhinitis is a reaction to airborne (inhaled) allergens. It's the most common atopic allergic reaction, affecting more than 20 million Americans. Rhinitis (inflammation of the nasal mucous membrane) and conjunctivitis (inflammation of the conjunctiva) may occur seasonally or year-round.

How it happens

Allergic rhinitis may occur from primary exposure or reexposure.

Primary exposure

During primary exposure to an allergen, T cells recognize the foreign allergens and release chemicals that instruct B cells to produce specific antibodies called *immunoglobulin E* (IgE). IgE antibodies attach themselves to mast cells. Mast cells with attached IgE can remain in the body for years, ready to react when they next encounter the same allergen.

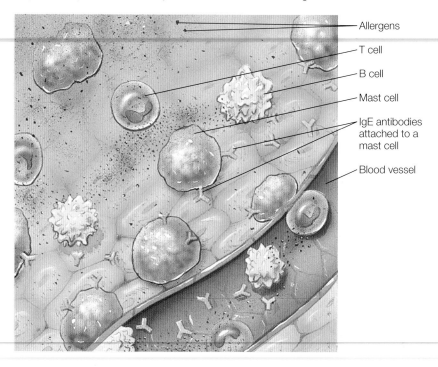

- Allergens
- T cell
- B cell
- Mast cell
- IgE antibodies attached to a mast cell
- Blood vessel

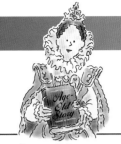

Age-old story

Age and allergic rhinitis

Allergic rhinitis is most prevalent in young children and adolescents but can occur in all age-groups.

What to look for

Seasonal

■ Paroxysmal sneezing; profuse, watery rhinorrhea (nasal mucus discharge); nasal obstruction or congestion; and itchy nose and eyes
■ Pale, cyanotic, edematous nasal mucosa
■ Red, edematous eyelids and conjunctivae
■ Excessive lacrimation
■ Headache or sinus pain
■ Itching in the throat and malaise
■ Dark circles under the eyes (allergic shiners)

Perennial

■ Conjunctivitis and other extranasal effects (rare)
■ Chronic nasal obstruction
■ Allergic shiners

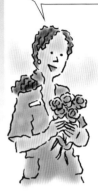

Roses are red, violets are blue, if I put these near me, I say "Achoo."

Reexposure

The second time the allergen enters the body, it comes into direct contact with the IgE antibodies attached to the mast cells. This contact stimulates the mast cells to release chemicals (such as histamine), which initiate a response that causes tightening of the smooth muscles in the airways, dilation of small blood vessels, increased mucus secretion in the nasal cavity and airways, and itching.

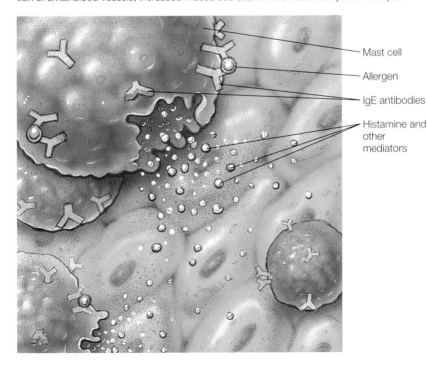

— Mast cell

— Allergen

— IgE antibodies

— Histamine and other mediators

Allergic shiners

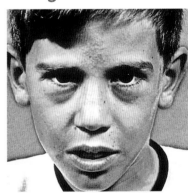

This photo shows mouth breathing and allergic shiners, a darkening of the intraorbital skin related to chronic nasal congestion.

Anaphylaxis

With prompt treatment, the prognosis for anaphylaxis is good. But a severe reaction may lead to systemic shock and sometimes death.

Anaphylaxis is an acute, potentially life-threatening type I (immediate) hypersensitivity reaction marked by the sudden onset of rapidly progressive urticaria (vascular swelling in the skin accompanied by itching) and respiratory distress. With prompt recognition and treatment, the prognosis is good. However, a severe reaction may precipitate vascular collapse, leading to systemic shock and, sometimes, death. The reaction typically occurs within minutes but can occur up to 1 hour after reexposure to the antigen.

How it happens

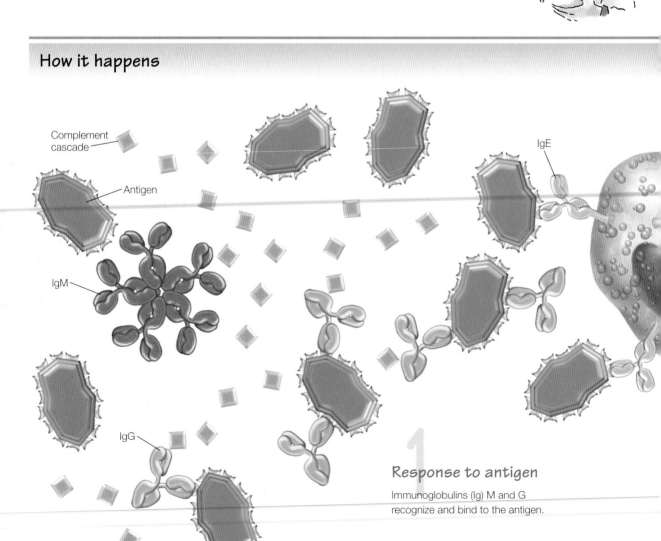

Complement cascade

Antigen

IgE

IgM

IgG

1 Response to antigen

Immunoglobulins (Ig) M and G recognize and bind to the antigen.

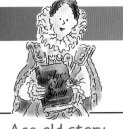

Age-old story

Age and anaphylaxis

Children are more likely to experience food-related anaphylaxis. Adults are more likely to experience anaphylaxis related to antibiotics, radiocontrast media, anesthetic agents, and insect stings.

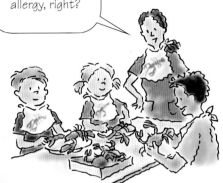

None of you kids has a seafood allergy, right?

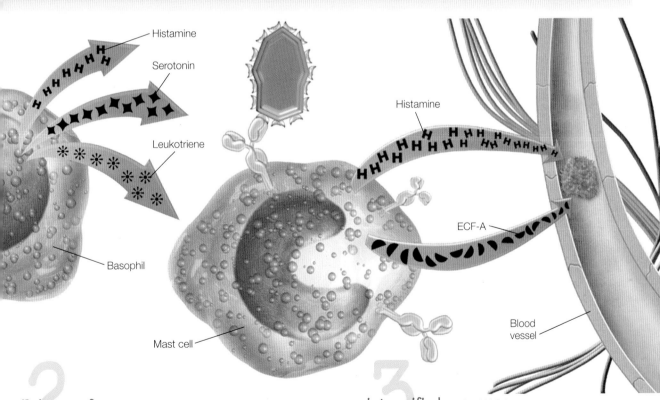

Histamine

Serotonin

Leukotriene

Basophil

Mast cell

Histamine

ECF-A

Blood vessel

Release of chemical mediators

Activated IgE on basophils promote the release of mediators: histamine, serotonin, and leukotrienes.

Intensified response

Mast cells release more histamine and ECF-A.

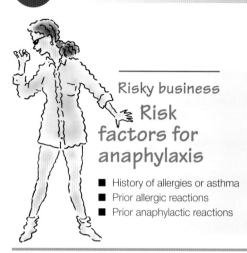

Risky business
Risk factors for anaphylaxis

- History of allergies or asthma
- Prior allergic reactions
- Prior anaphylactic reactions

What to look for

Initial

- Feeling of impending doom or fright
- Sweating
- Shortness of breath
- Nasal pruritus
- Urticaria
- Angioedema

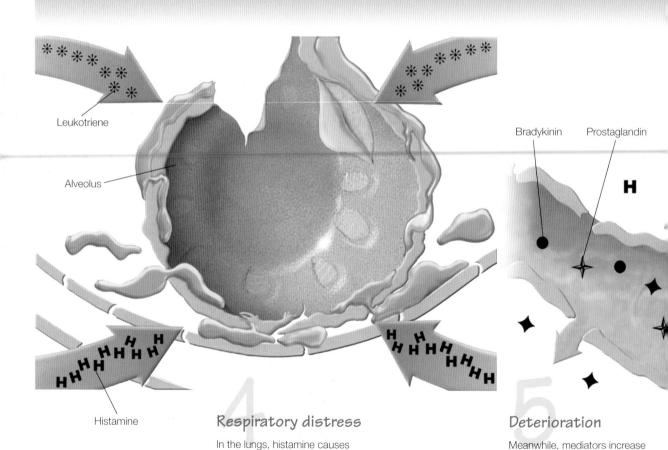

Leukotriene

Alveolus

Bradykinin   Prostaglandin

H

Histamine

4 Respiratory distress

In the lungs, histamine causes endothelial cell destruction and fluid to leak into alveoli.

5 Deterioration

Meanwhile, mediators increase vascular permeability, causing fluid to leak from the vessels.

Systemic

■ Hypotension, shock, and sometimes cardiac arrhythmias
■ Nasal mucosal edema; profuse, watery rhinorrhea; itching; nasal congestion; and sudden sneezing attacks
■ Edema of the upper respiratory tract, resulting in hypopharyngeal and laryngeal obstruction
■ Hoarseness, stridor, wheezing, and accessory muscle use
■ Severe stomach cramps, nausea, diarrhea, and urinary urgency and incontinence

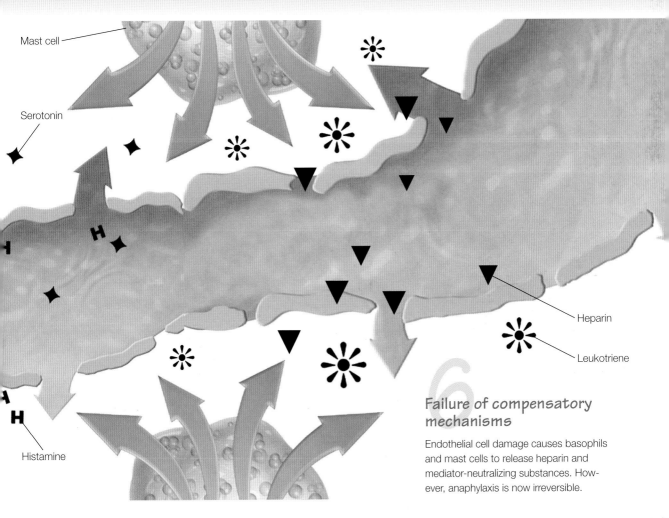

Mast cell

Serotonin

Heparin

Leukotriene

Histamine

6 Failure of compensatory mechanisms

Endothelial cell damage causes basophils and mast cells to release heparin and mediator-neutralizing substances. However, anaphylaxis is now irreversible.

Ankylosing spondylitis

Ankylosing spondylitis is a chronic, usually progressive inflammatory bone disease that primarily affects the sacroiliac, apophyseal, and costovertebral joints along with the adjacent soft tissue. The disease, also known as *rheumatoid spondylitis* and *Marie-Strümpell disease*, usually begins in the sacroiliac joints and gradually progresses to the lumbar, thoracic, and cervical regions of the spine. Deterioration of the bone and cartilage can lead to formation of fibrous tissue and eventual fusion of the spine or the peripheral joints.

How it happens

Fibrous tissue of the joint capsule is infiltrated by inflammatory cells that erode the bone and fibrocartilage. Repair of the cartilaginous structures begins with the proliferation of fibroblasts, which synthesize and secrete collagen. The collagen forms fibrous scar tissue that eventually undergoes calcification and ossification, causing the joint to fuse or lose flexibility. The result is ultimate destruction of these joints with fusion of the spine. The vertebrae have a squared appearance and bone bridges fuse one vertebral body to the next across the intervertebral disks.

> Ankylosing spondylitis usually begins in the sacroiliac joints and progresses to the lumbar, thoracic, and cervical regions of the spine.

Spinal fusion in ankylosing spondylitis

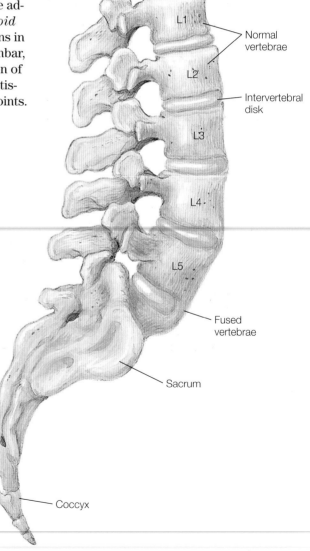

Normal vertebrae

Intervertebral disk

L1

L2

L3

L4

L5

Fused vertebrae

Sacrum

Coccyx

Lateral view

A closer look

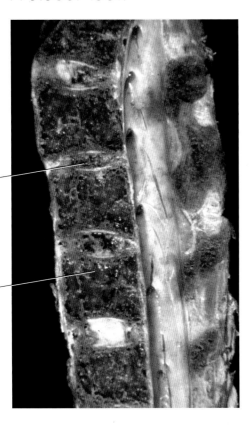

Intervertebral disk replaced by marrow

Osteoporosis from disease

What to look for

■ Intermittent low back pain (more severe in the morning or after inactivity and relieved by exercise)
■ Mild fatigue, fever, anorexia, weight loss
■ Pain in the shoulders, hips, knees, and ankles
■ Pain over the symphysis pubis
■ Stiffness or limited motion of the lumbar spine
■ Warmth, swelling, or tenderness of the affected joints

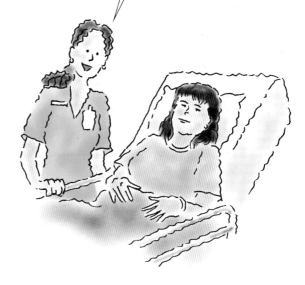

Pain in the lower back, shoulders, hips, knees, and ankles? Ankylosing spondylitis might be the culprit!

Atopic dermatitis

Atopic dermatitis, also referred to as *eczema*, is a chronic skin disorder characterized by superficial skin inflammation and intense pruritus (itching). Although this disorder may appear at any age, it typically begins during infancy or early childhood. It may then subside spontaneously, followed by exacerbations in late childhood, adolescence, or early adulthood.

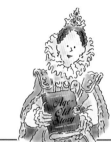

Age-old story

Age and atopic dermatitis

About 10% of childhood cases of atopic dermatitis are caused by allergy to certain foods, especially eggs, milk, peanuts, and wheat.

While atopic dermatitis affects less than 1% of the population, for those it does affect, it causes intense itching.

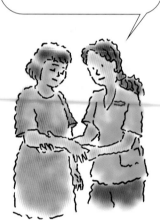

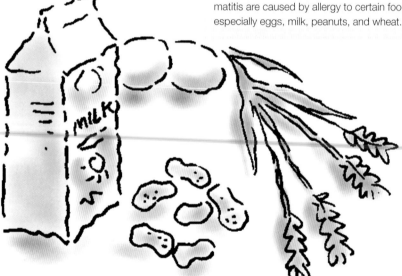

How it happens

In atopic dermatitis, the allergic mechanism of hypersensitivity results in a release of inflammatory mediators through sensitized antibodies of the IgE class. Histamine and other cytokines induce acute inflammation. Abnormally dry skin and a decreased threshold for itching set up the "itch-scratch-itch" cycle, which eventually causes lesions (excoriations, lichenification).

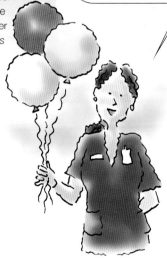

Risky business
Risk factors for atopic dermatitis

- *Genetic factors*—greater chance of atopic dermatitis in children whose parents have allergic disorders
- *Environmental factors*—skin irritants, including wool or synthetic clothing, soaps or detergents, cosmetics or perfumes, dust and sand, chemical solvents, and chlorine; extremes in temperature or climate; and lack of moisturizing after bathing
- *Medical conditions*—allergies to plant pollen, animal dander, household dust mites, molds, and certain foods

A closer look

The top photo shows atopic dermatitis in an infant; the bottom one shows atopic dermatitis in an adult.

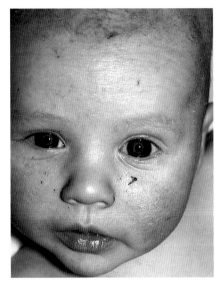

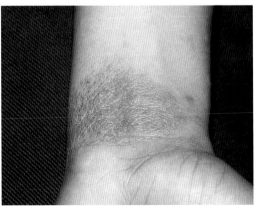

What to look for

- Erythematous, weeping lesions
- Scaling and lichenification of lesions
- In children: characteristic pink pigmentation and swelling of the upper eyelid and a double fold under the lower lid, called *Morgan's line* or *Dennie's sign*

> These signs and symptoms make me think of yellow for weeping lesions, red for scaling lesions, and pink for pink pigmentation and swelling of the eyelids.

Rheumatoid arthritis

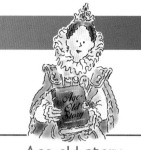

Age-old story

Age and RA

RA can occur at any age but the peak onset is ages 30 to 60. Life expectancy for a person with RA may be shortened by an average of about 5 years.

Rheumatoid arthritis (RA) is a chronic, systemic inflammatory disease that primarily attacks peripheral joints and the surrounding muscles, tendons, ligaments, and blood vessels. Partial remissions and unpredictable exacerbations mark the course of this potentially crippling disease.

RA is three times more common in women than men. It occurs worldwide, affecting more than 2.1 million people in the United States alone.

How it happens

The cause of RA isn't known, but infections, genetics, and endocrine factors may play a part.

When exposed to an antigen, a person susceptible to RA may develop abnormal or altered IgG antibodies. The body doesn't recognize these antibodies as "self," so it forms an antibody, known as *rheumatoid factor,* against them. By aggregating into complexes, rheumatoid factor causes inflammation.

Eventually, inflammation causes cartilage damage. Immune responses continue, including complement system activation. Complement system activation attracts leukocytes and stimulates the release of inflammatory mediators, which then exacerbate joint destruction.

Four stages of inflammation

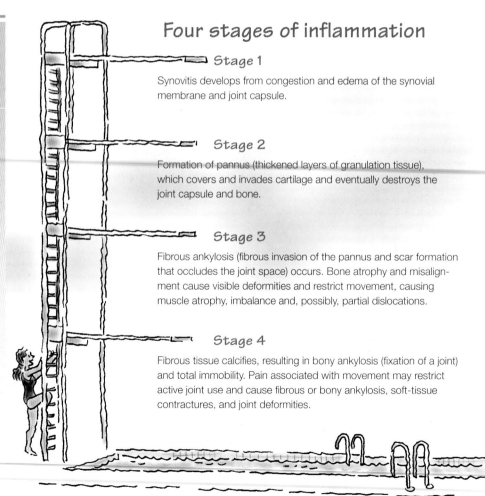

Stage 1
Synovitis develops from congestion and edema of the synovial membrane and joint capsule.

Stage 2
Formation of pannus (thickened layers of granulation tissue), which covers and invades cartilage and eventually destroys the joint capsule and bone.

Stage 3
Fibrous ankylosis (fibrous invasion of the pannus and scar formation that occludes the joint space) occurs. Bone atrophy and misalignment cause visible deformities and restrict movement, causing muscle atrophy, imbalance and, possibly, partial dislocations.

Stage 4
Fibrous tissue calcifies, resulting in bony ankylosis (fixation of a joint) and total immobility. Pain associated with movement may restrict active joint use and cause fibrous or bony ankylosis, soft-tissue contractures, and joint deformities.

Effects of RA on certain joints

Hand and wrist

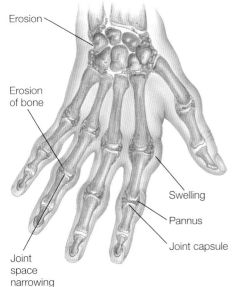

Erosion

Erosion of bone

Joint space narrowing

Swelling

Pannus

Joint capsule

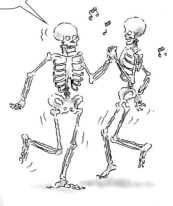

...you put your right hand in and ya shake it all about...

Knee

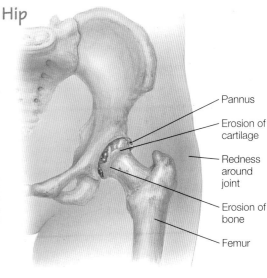

Erosion of cartilage

Erosion of bone

Pannus covering synovial membrane

memory board

Synovitis develops.

Pannis forms.

Ankylosis (fibrous) occurs.

Tissue calcifies.

No, I didn't say, "Spam." I said "SPAT" is the way to remember the four stages of RA.

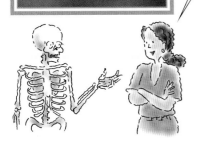

What to look for

- Fatigue
- Malaise
- Anorexia
- Persistent low-grade fever
- Weight loss
- Vague articular symptoms

Hip

Pannus

Erosion of cartilage

Redness around joint

Erosion of bone

Femur

VISION QUEST

Photo finish

Number these illustrations (1 to 6) in the correct order as to how anaphylaxis develops.

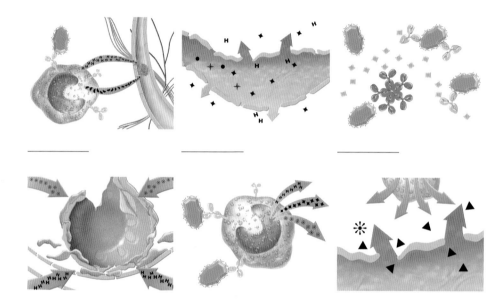

Rebus riddle

Solve the riddle to learn a characteristic of a skin disorder.

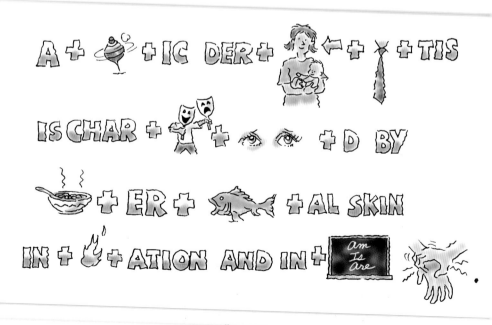

9 Endocrine disorders

Did somebody say, "Graves' disease?" This chapter and this pirate role seem to go hand-in-hand!

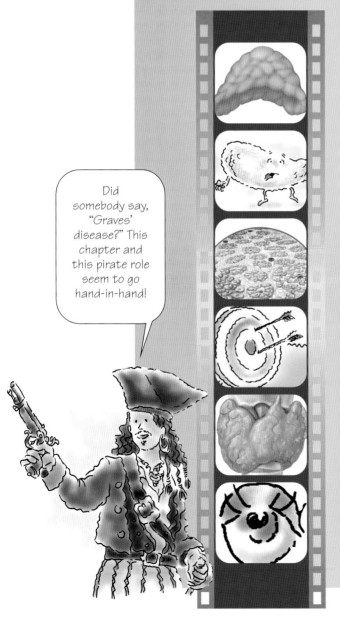

Adrenal hypofunction

Adrenal hypofunction occurs in two forms: primary and secondary. Both forms can progress into adrenal crisis.

Primary

Primary adrenal hypofunction or insufficiency (also called *Addison's disease*) originates within the adrenal gland and is characterized by the decreased secretion of mineralocorticoids, glucocorticoids, and androgens. Addison's disease is relatively uncommon and can occur at any age and in both genders.

Secondary

The secondary form of adrenal hypofunction is caused by a disorder outside the gland, such as a pituitary tumor with corticotropin deficiency, or abrupt withdrawal of long-term corticosteroid therapy. In secondary forms of the disorder, aldosterone secretion may be unaffected.

How it happens

In Addison's disease, more than 90% of both adrenal glands are destroyed. Massive destruction usually results from an autoimmune process whereby circulating antibodies attack adrenal tissue. This leads to a rapid decline in the steroid hormones cortisol and aldosterone, which directly affects the liver, stomach, and kidneys.

Adrenal crisis

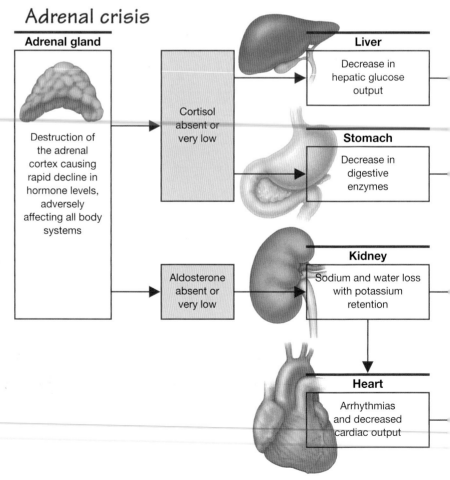

Adrenal gland

Destruction of the adrenal cortex causing rapid decline in hormone levels, adversely affecting all body systems

Cortisol absent or very low

Aldosterone absent or very low

Liver
Decrease in hepatic glucose output

Stomach
Decrease in digestive enzymes

Kidney
Sodium and water loss with potassium retention

Heart
Arrhythmias and decreased cardiac output

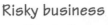

Risky business
Risk factors for adrenal crisis

Adrenal crisis usually develops in patients who:
- don't respond to hormone replacement therapy
- experience extreme stress without adequate glucocorticoid replacement
- abruptly stop hormone therapy
- experience trauma
- undergo bilateral adrenalectomy.

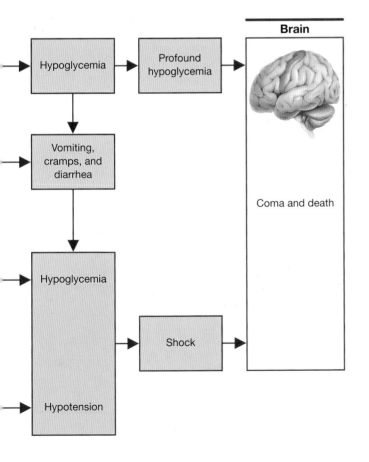

Brain

Hypoglycemia → Profound hypoglycemia →

Vomiting, cramps, and diarrhea

Hypoglycemia

Shock →

Hypotension

Coma and death

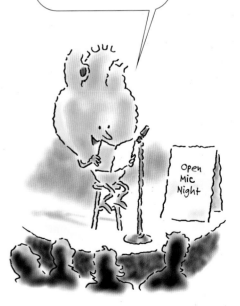

Adrenal crisis and hypotension... Know how it happens and you learn your lesson!

Open Mic Night

Blocked secretion of cortisol in primary adrenal hypofunction

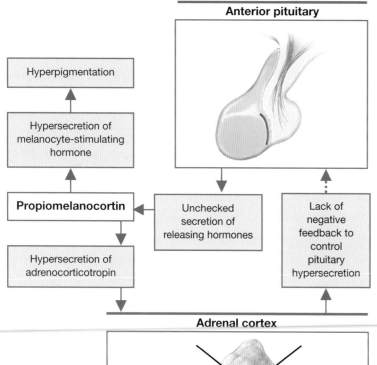

Anterior pituitary

Hyperpigmentation

↑

Hypersecretion of melanocyte-stimulating hormone

↑

Propiomelanocortin ← Unchecked secretion of releasing hormones

Lack of negative feedback to control pituitary hypersecretion

↓

Hypersecretion of adrenocorticotropin

Adrenal cortex

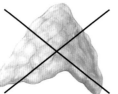

Hypofunction of adrenal cortex, resulting in insufficient production of cortisol

What to look for

Primary

- Weakness and fatigue
- Weight loss, nausea, vomiting, and anorexia
- Conspicuous bronze color of the skin, especially in the creases of the hands and over the metacarpophalangeal joints (hand and finger), elbows, and knees
- Darkening of scars, areas of vitiligo (absence of pigmentation), and increased pigmentation of the mucous membranes, especially the buccal mucosa
- Orthostatic hypotension, decreased cardiac size and output, and weak, irregular pulse
- Decreased tolerance for even minor stress
- Fasting hypoglycemia
- Craving salty food

Secondary

- Similar to primary but without hyperpigmentation
- Possibly no hypotension and electrolyte abnormalities
- Usually normal androgen secretion

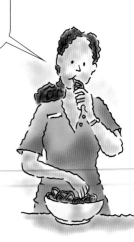

These pretzels are making me thirsty! But I just crave salty foods!

Diabetes mellitus

Diabetes mellitus is a disease in which the body doesn't produce or properly use insulin, leading to hyperglycemia.

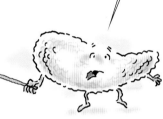

Diabetes mellitus occurs in two primary forms.

1. Type 1 (formerly called *insulin-dependent diabetes mellitus*)

2. Type 2 (formerly called *non-insulin-dependent diabetes mellitus*), the more prevalent form

Several secondary forms also exist, caused by such conditions as pancreatic disease, pregnancy (gestational diabetes mellitus), hormonal or genetic problems, and certain drugs or chemicals.

How it happens

Normally, insulin allows glucose to travel into cells. There, it's used for energy and stored as glycogen. Insulin also stimulates protein synthesis and free fatty acid storage in adipose tissue. Insulin deficiency blocks tissues' access to essential nutrients for fuel and storage. The pathophysiology behind each type of diabetes differs.

Type 1 diabetes
■ Pancreas makes little or no insulin.
■ In genetically susceptible patients, a triggering event (possibly a viral infection) causes production of autoantibodies against the beta cells of the pancreas.
■ Resultant destruction of beta cells leads to a decline in and ultimate lack of insulin secretion.
■ Insulin deficiency leads to hyperglycemia, enhanced lipolysis (fat breakdown), and protein catabolism. These conditions occur when more than 90% of the beta cells have been destroyed.

Type 2 diabetes
■ Genetic factors are significant.
■ Onset is accelerated by obesity and a sedentary lifestyle.
■ The pancreas produces some insulin, but it's either too little or ineffective.
■ Impaired glucose secretion, inappropriate hepatic glucose production, and peripheral insulin receptor insensitivity contribute to its development.

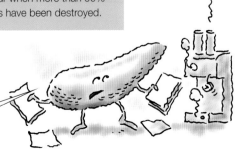

It figures! I've got all these orders for insulin and my Insulin-o-matic is broken.

Understanding type 2 diabetes

Normally, in response to blood glucose levels, the pancreatic islets of Langerhans release insulin. In type 2 diabetes, problems arise when insufficient insulin is produced or when the body's cells resist insulin.

Normal insulin-producing pancreatic islet of Langerhans

Diabetic islet of Langerhans

Cellular view of the pancreas

Glucose molecule (from digestive system)

Insulin molecule (from pancreas)

Red blood cell

Normal body cell

Normally, insulin molecules bind to the preceptors on the body's cells. When activated by insulin, portals open to allow glucose to enter the cell, where it's converted to energy.

Diabetic body cell

In type 2 diabetes, the body's cells develop a resistance to insulin, making it more difficult for glucose to enter the cell.

Opened glucose portal

Closed glucose portal

Insulin receptor

Glucose converted to energy

Energy-deprived cell

As a result, cells don't get enough energy. This lack of energy causes glucose to build up in the blood vessels, resulting in damage to all body organs.

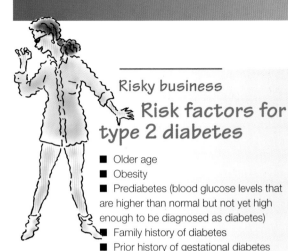

Risky business

Risk factors for type 2 diabetes

- Older age
- Obesity
- Prediabetes (blood glucose levels that are higher than normal but not yet high enough to be diagnosed as diabetes)
- Family history of diabetes
- Prior history of gestational diabetes
- Race or ethnicity (Blacks, Hispanics, Native Americans, and Asians)

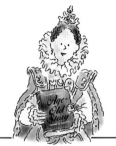

Age-old story

Age and diabetes

Type 1 diabetes is the most common form of diabetes in children. Symptoms that are more typical for children include:

- stomach pains
- headaches
- behavior problems.

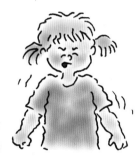

NO! My stomach doesn't hurt. NO! I don't have a headache! NO! You're not going to stick me with that needle.

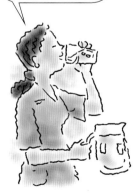

I just can't get enough of this stuff.

What to look for

Type 1 diabetes
- Extreme thirst
- High levels of ketones in urine
- Lack of or increase in appetite
- Drowsiness, lethargy
- Fruity odor to breath
- Frequent urination
- High glucose levels in blood or urine
- Rapid, hard, or heavy breathing
- Eventual stupor to unconsciousness

Type 2 diabetes
- Possibly produces no symptoms
- Frequent urination
- Excessive thirst
- Fatigue
- Very dry skin
- Sores that are slow to heal
- More infections than usual
- Tingling or numbness in the hands
- Dehydration
- Unexplained weight loss
- Extreme hunger
- Sudden vision change

Hyperthyroidism

An overproduction of thyroid hormone creates a metabolic imbalance called *hyperthyroidism* or *thyrotoxicosis*. Excess thyroid hormone can cause various thyroid disorders; Graves' disease is the most common.

How it happens

In Graves' disease, thyroid-stimulating antibodies bind to and stimulate the thyroid-stimulating hormone (TSH) receptors of the thyroid gland.

The trigger for this autoimmune response is unclear; it may have several causes. Genetic factors may play a part because the disease tends to occur in identical twins. Immunologic factors may also be the culprit. The disease occasionally coexists with other autoimmune endocrine abnormalities, such as type 1 diabetes mellitus, thyroiditis, and hyperparathyroidism.

> I feel grave. Actually, Graves' disease is an autoimmune disorder that causes goiter and multiple systemic changes.

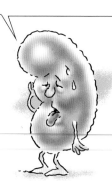

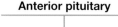
Anterior pituitary

↓

T-cell lymphocytes become sensitized to thyroid antigens.

↓

T-cell lymphocytes stimulate B-cell lymphocytes to secrete autoantibodies.

↓

Thyroid gland

Thyroid-stimulating antibodies bind to and stimulate TSH receptors of the thyroid gland.

↓

Increased production of thyroid hormones and cell growth result.

What to look for

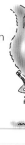

When onset follows physical or emotional stress
- Enlarged thyroid gland
- Exophthalmos (abnormal protrusion of the eye)
- Nervousness
- Heat intolerance
- Weight loss despite increased appetite
- Excessive sweating
- Diarrhea
- Tremors
- Palpitations
- Others due to thyroid hormone effects on all body systems

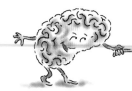

Central nervous system
- Most common in younger patients
- Difficulty concentrating
- Anxiety
- Excitability or nervousness, fine tremor, shaky handwriting, clumsiness, emotional instability, and mood swings ranging from occasional outbursts to overt psychosis

Cardiovascular system
- Most common in elderly patients
- Arrhythmias, especially atrial fibrillation
- Cardiac insufficiency
- Cardiac decompensation
- Resistance to the usual therapeutic dosage of digoxin

Integumentary system

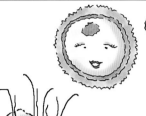
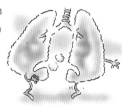

- Vitiligo and skin hyperpigmentation
- Warm, moist, flushed skin with a velvety texture
- Fine, soft hair
- Premature graying
- Hair loss in both sexes
- Fragile nails
- Onycholysis (separation of distal nail from nail bed)
- Pretibial myxedema producing raised, thickened skin and plaquelike or nodular lesions

Reproductive system

- Menstrual abnormalities
- Impaired fertility
- Decreased libido
- Gynecomastia (abnormal development of mammary glands in men)

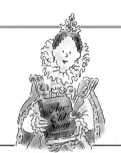

Age-old story

Age and Graves' disease

The incidence of Graves' disease is greatest in women between ages 30 and 60, especially those with a family history of thyroid abnormalities.

Only 5% of patients with Graves' disease are younger than age 15.

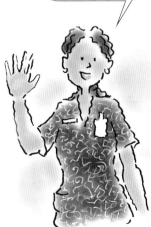

Respiratory system

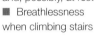
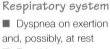

- Dyspnea on exertion and, possibly, at rest
- Breathlessness when climbing stairs

Eyes

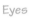

- Infrequent blinking
- Lid lag
- Reddened conjunctiva and cornea
- Corneal ulcers
- Impaired upward gaze
- Convergence (turning the eyes in)
- Strabismus (eye deviation)
- Exophthalmos

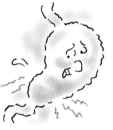

GI system

- Anorexia
- Nausea and vomiting

Graves' disease symptoms

This photo shows the major symptoms of Graves' disease: exophthalmos and goiter.

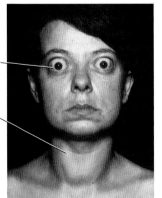

Musculoskeletal system

- Muscle weakness
- Generalized or localized muscle atrophy
- Acropachy (soft-tissue swelling with underlying bone changes where new bone formation occurs)
- Osteoporosis

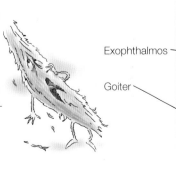

Exophthalmos

Goiter

Hypothyroidism

In hypothyroidism (thyroid hormone deficiency) in adults, metabolic processes slow down. This slowing is caused by a deficit in triiodothyronine (T_3) or thyroxine (T_4), both of which regulate metabolism.

Hypothyroidism is classified as *primary* or *secondary*. The primary form stems from a disorder of the thyroid gland itself. The secondary form stems from a failure to stimulate normal thyroid function.

> The secondary form of hypothyroidism may progress to myxedema coma, a medical emergency.

What to look for

Early

- Energy loss
- Fatigue
- Forgetfulness
- Sensitivity to cold
- Unexplained weight gain
- Constipation

Progressive

- Anorexia
- Decreased libido
- Menorrhagia (painful menstruation)
- Paresthesia (numbness, prickling, or tingling)
- Joint stiffness
- Muscle cramping

How it happens

Primary

- Thyroidectomy
- Inflammation from radiation therapy
- Other inflammatory conditions, such as amyloidosis and sarcoidosis
- Chronic autoimmune thyroiditis (Hashimoto's disease)

Secondary

- Failure to stimulate normal thyroid function (For example, the pituitary may fail to produce thyroid-stimulating hormone [TSH] [thyrotropin] or the hypothalamus may fail to produce thyrotropin-releasing hormone [TRH].)
- Inability to synthesize thyroid hormones due to iodine deficiency (usually dietary) or the use of antithyroid medications

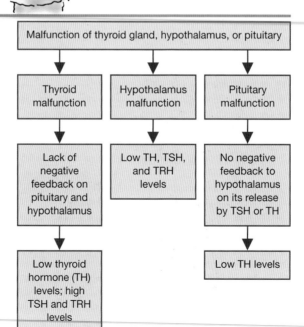

Malfunction of thyroid gland, hypothalamus, or pituitary

Thyroid malfunction → Lack of negative feedback on pituitary and hypothalamus → Low thyroid hormone (TH) levels; high TSH and TRH levels

Hypothalamus malfunction → Low TH, TSH, and TRH levels

Pituitary malfunction → No negative feedback to hypothalamus on its release by TSH or TH → Low TH levels

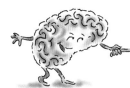

Central nervous system

- Psychiatric disturbances
- Ataxia (loss of coordination)
- Intention tremor (tremor during voluntary motion)
- Carpal tunnel syndrome
- Benign intracranial hypertension
- Behavioral changes ranging from slight mental slowing to severe impairment

Cardiovascular system

- Hypercholesterolemia (high cholesterol) with associated arteriosclerosis and ischemic heart disease
- Poor peripheral circulation
- Heart enlargement
- Heart failure
- Pleural and pericardial effusions

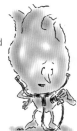

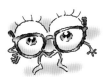

Eyes and ears

- Conductive or sensorineural deafness and nystagmus

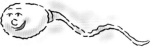

GI system

- Achlorhydria (absence of free hydrochloric acid in the stomach)
- Pernicious anemia
- Adynamic (weak) colon, resulting in megacolon (extremely dilated colon) and intestinal obstruction

Integumentary system

- Dry, flaky, inelastic skin
- Puffy face, hands, and feet
- Dry, sparse hair with patchy hair loss and loss of the outer third of the eyebrow
- Thick, brittle nails with transverse and longitudinal grooves
- Thick, dry tongue, causing hoarseness and slow, slurred speech

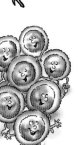

Reproductive system

- Impaired fertility

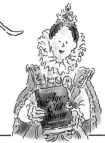

Hematologic system

- Anemia, possibly resulting in bleeding tendencies and iron deficiency anemia

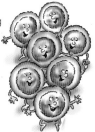

Age-old story

Age and hypothyroidism

Hypothyroidism occurs primarily after age 40. In fact, 10% of all women older than age 50 show signs of a failing thyroid, as opposed to 3% of men older than age 50.

Metabolic syndrome

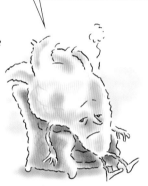

A metabolic syndrome diagnosis raises a person's risk of heart disease and stroke and places him at high risk for dying of a myocardial infarction.

Metabolic syndrome—also called *syndrome X, insulin resistance syndrome, dysmetabolic syndrome,* or *multiple metabolic syndrome*—is a cluster of conditions characterized by:
- abdominal obesity
- high blood glucose level (type 2 diabetes mellitus)
- insulin resistance
- high blood cholesterol and triglyceride levels
- high blood pressure.

More than 22% of people in the United States demonstrate three or more of these characteristics, meeting the requirements for a diagnosis of metabolic syndrome.

How it happens

In the normal digestion process, the intestines break down food into its basic components, one of which is glucose. Glucose provides energy for cellular activity, and excess glucose is stored in cells for future use. Insulin, a hormone secreted in the pancreas, guides glucose into storage cells.

However, in people with metabolic syndrome, glucose is insulin-resistant and doesn't respond to insulin's attempt to guide it into storage cells. Excess insulin is then required to overcome this resistance. This excess in quantity and force of insulin causes damage to the lining of the arteries, promotes fat storage deposits, and prevents fat breakdown. This series of events can lead to diabetes, blood clots, and coronary events.

Effects of metabolic syndrome

Organs affected by metabolic syndrome

Brain

Pancreas

Heart

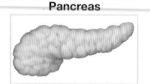

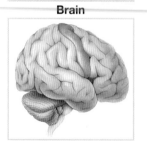

No way, man. You aren't the boss of me!

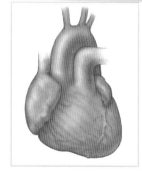

Fibrous plaque (atherosclerosis)

What to look for

Symptom: Abdominal obesity (evidenced by a waist of more than 40" [101.6 cm] in men and 35" [88.9 cm] in women) caused by poor diet and sedentary lifestyle.

Symptom: Blood pressure of 130/85 mm Hg or higher due to a history of hypertension.

Symptom: Fasting blood glucose level of 100 mg/dl or higher due to diabetes or prediabetes.

High blood glucose
Glucose builds up in the bloodstream.

High blood pressure
If untreated, damage to the lining of the arteries results.

Fibrous plaque
Elevated cholesterol levels lead to fibrous deposits in the blood vessels.

Risky business
Risk factors for metabolic syndrome

The American Heart Association has determined that a patient with three or more of these factors is at risk for developing metabolic syndrome:
- elevated waist circumference—40" (101.6 cm) or more in men; 35" (88.9 cm) or more in women
- elevated triglyceride level—150 mg/dl or higher
- reduced HDL ("good") cholesterol—less than 40 mg/dl in men; less than 50 mg/dl in women
- elevated blood pressure—130/85 mm Hg or higher
- elevated fasting glucose level—100 mg/dl or higher.

SIADH

The syndrome of inappropriate antidiuretic hormone secretion (SIADH) results when excessive antidiuretic hormone (ADH) secretion is triggered by stimuli other than increased extracellular fluid osmolarity and decreased extracellular fluid volume, reflected by hypotension. SIADH is a relatively common complication of surgery or critical illness. It may develop in some children during the acute phase of meningitis. The prognosis varies with the degree of disease and the speed at which it develops. SIADH usually resolves within 3 days of effective treatment.

What to look for

- Fatigue, lethargy, anorexia, and thirst (first signs and symptoms)
- Vomiting
- Intestinal cramping
- Weight gain
- Edema
- Water retention
- Decreased urine output
- Restlessness
- Confusion
- Headache
- Irritability
- Seizures
- Coma
- Decreased deep tendon reflexes

How it happens

In the presence of excessive ADH, excessive water reabsorption from the distal convoluted tubule and collecting ducts causes hyponatremia and normal to slightly increased extracellular fluid volume.

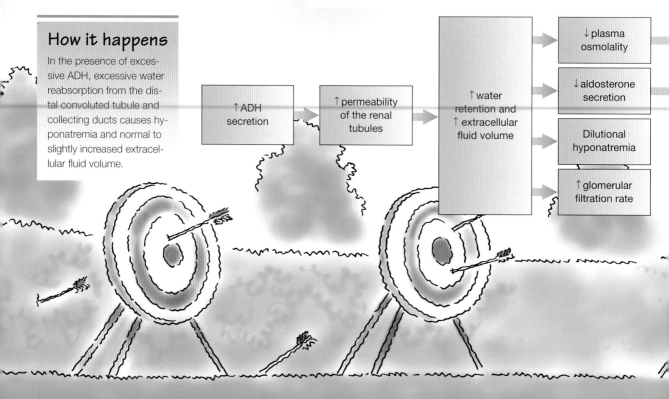

↑ADH secretion → ↑permeability of the renal tubules → ↑water retention and ↑extracellular fluid volume → ↓plasma osmolality / ↓aldosterone secretion / Dilutional hyponatremia / ↑glomerular filtration rate

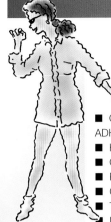

Risky business
Risk factors for SIADH

- Oat-cell or small-cell lung cancer (secretes excessive ADH), pancreatic or prostate cancer
- Hodgkin's disease
- Central nervous system disorders
- Pulmonary disorders
- Certain drugs
- Thymomas
- Myxedema
- Psychosis

Sing out—in A FLAT—to remember the first symptoms that appear in SIADH.

memory board

Fatigue

Lethargy

Anorexia

Thirst

↑sodium excretion and a shifting of fluid into cells

Patient develops thirst, dyspnea on exertion, vomiting, abdominal cramps, confusion, lethargy, and hyponatremia.

Follow the arrows to find out what happens in SIADH.

Thyroid cancer

Thyroid cancer (also called *thyroid carcinoma*) is the most common endocrine malignancy. It occurs in all age-groups, especially in people who have undergone radiation treatment of the neck area. There are three main types:

 papillary

 follicular

medullary.

How it happens

Papillary carcinoma accounts for one-half of all thyroid cancers in adults. Most common in young females, it's the least virulent form of thyroid cancer and metastasizes slowly.

Follicular carcinoma is less common but more likely to recur and metastasize to the regional lymph nodes and through blood vessels into the bones, liver, and lungs.

Medullary carcinoma originates in the parafollicular cells and contains amyloid and calcium deposits. It can produce thyrocalcitonin, histamine, adrenocorticotropin (producing Cushing's syndrome), and prostaglandin E_2 and F_3 (producing diarrhea). This rare form of thyroid cancer is familial, associated with pheochromocytoma, and completely curable when detected before it causes symptoms. Untreated, it progresses rapidly. Seldom curable by resection, these tumors resist radiation and metastasize quickly.

Early, localized thyroid cancer

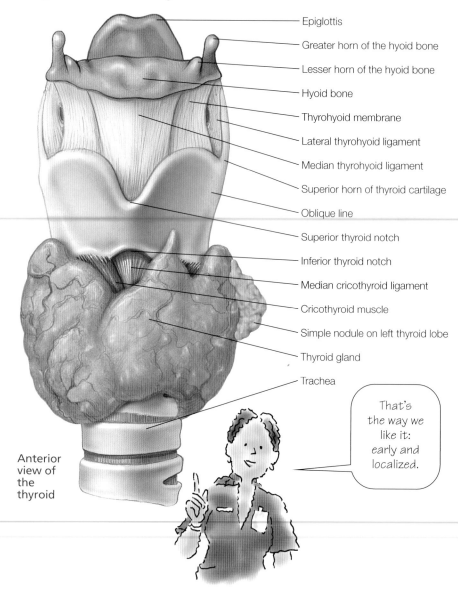

- Epiglottis
- Greater horn of the hyoid bone
- Lesser horn of the hyoid bone
- Hyoid bone
- Thyrohyoid membrane
- Lateral thyrohyoid ligament
- Median thyrohyoid ligament
- Superior horn of thyroid cartilage
- Oblique line
- Superior thyroid notch
- Inferior thyroid notch
- Median cricothyroid ligament
- Cricothyroid muscle
- Simple nodule on left thyroid lobe
- Thyroid gland
- Trachea

Anterior view of the thyroid

That's the way we like it: early and localized.

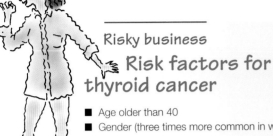

Risky business
Risk factors for thyroid cancer

- Age older than 40
- Gender (three times more common in women than men)
- Race (more common in Whites than Blacks)
- Iodine deficiency
- Radiation exposure
- High-dose X-rays
- Heredity (family history of thyroid cancer, goiter, or colon polyps)

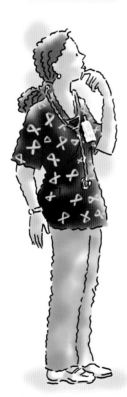

What to look for

- Painless nodule, hard nodule in an enlarged thyroid gland, or palpable lymph nodes and thyroid enlargement
- Cough
- Hoarseness, dysphagia, and pain on palpation
- Hypothyroidism (low metabolism, mental apathy, sensitivity to cold) or hyperthyroidism (hyperactivity, restlessness, sensitivity to heat)
- Diarrhea, anorexia, irritability, vocal cord paralysis.

Papillary carcinoma of the thyroid

This photograph shows a resected thyroid gland with a beige mass, which is papillary carcinoma.

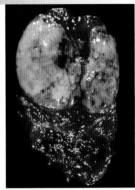

Follicular adenoma

This photograph shows an encapsulated mass of follicular adenoma with hemorrhage, fibrosis, and cystic changes.

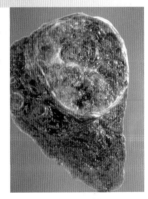

Medullary thyroid carcinoma

This photograph shows a section of a thyroid resection with a pale tumor, indicating medullary carcinoma.

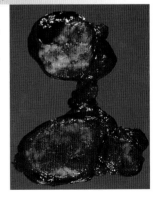

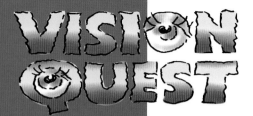

My word!

Solve the word scrambles to discover four major signs and symptoms of diabetes mellitus. Then rearrange the circled letters from those words to answer the question posed.

Question: What is a major component of diabetes mellitus?

1. remxtee stthri _ _ _ _ _ _ _ _   _ _○_○

2. gutifae _ _ _ _ _ _○

3. reqenutf naonruiti

_ _ _ _ _ _○_   _ _ _ _ _ _ _○

4. redltae ppttaeie

_○_ _ _ _ _   _ _ _ _ _○_ _

Answer: _ _ _ _ _ _ _ _

Show and tell

Identify the two signs of Graves' disease pictured in this photo and explain their importance.

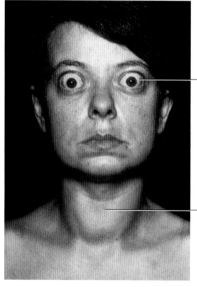

1. _____
_____
_____
_____

2. _____
_____
_____
_____

10
Renal disorders

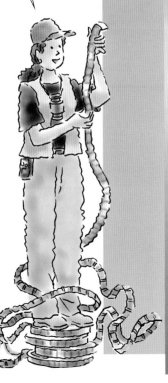

Monitoring renal disorders is crucial. So is monitoring how much film you've used. Has anyone seen the close-up shot of the kidney in the hospital?

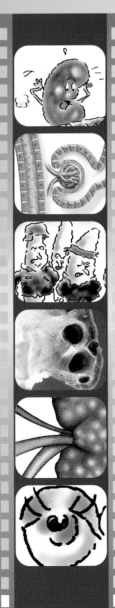

Acute renal failure

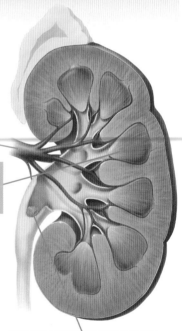

Oh no! An interruption in my work flow! This can lead to serious failure!

Acute renal failure is the sudden interruption of renal function. It can be caused by obstruction, poor circulation, or kidney disease. It's potentially reversible; however, if left untreated, permanent damage can lead to chronic renal failure.

How it happens

Acute renal failure may be classified as prerenal, intrarenal, or postrenal. Each type has separate causes.

Mechanism of acute renal failure

Prerenal failure
(marked decrease in renal blood flow)

- Antihypertensives
- Arrhythmias that cause reduced cardiac output
- Arterial embolism
- Arterial or venous thrombosis
- Ascites
- Burns
- Cardiac tamponade
- Cardiogenic shock
- Dehydration
- Disseminated intravascular coagulation
- Diuretic overuse
- Eclampsia
- Heart failure
- Hemorrhage
- Hypoalbuminemia
- Hypovolemic shock
- Malignant hypertension
- Myocardial infarction
- Pulmonary embolism
- Sepsis
- Trauma
- Tumor
- Vasculitis

Intrarenal failure
(damage to the structures of the kidney)

- Acute glomerulonephritis
- Acute tubular necrosis
- Acute pyelonephritis
- Bilateral renal vein thrombosis
- Crush injuries
- Malignant nephrosclerosis
- Myopathy
- Nephrotoxins
- Obstetric complications
- Papillary necrosis
- Polyarteritis nodosa
- Poorly treated prerenal failure
- Renal myeloma
- Scleroderma
- Sickle cell disease
- Systemic lupus erythematosus
- Transfusion reaction
- Vasculitis

Postrenal failure
(obstruction of urine outflow from kidney [renal calculi])

- Bladder obstruction
- Prostatic hypertrophy
- Ureteral obstruction
- Urethral obstruction

Phases of acute renal failure

The three types of acute renal failure (prerenal, intrarenal, and postrenal) usually include three distinct phases: oliguric, diuretic, and recovery.

What to look for

Acute renal failure is a critical illness. Its early signs and symptoms are oliguria (decreased urine output), azotemia (excess levels of urea in blood) and, rarely, anuria (failure to secrete urine). Electrolyte imbalance, metabolic acidosis, and other severe effects follow as the patient becomes increasingly uremic and renal dysfunction disrupts other body systems.

Oliguric phase

- Decreased urine output of less than 400 ml/24 hours (oliguria)

▼

- Decreased blood flow to the kidney (prerenal oliguria)

▼

- Impairment of kidney's ability to conserve sodium

▼

- Acute tubular necrosis possibly resulting from prerenal oliguria

▼

- Increased blood urea nitrogen (BUN) and creatinine levels and decreased ratio of BUN to creatinine (from normal levels of 20:1 to abnormal decrease of 10:1)

▼

- Hypervolemia

▼

- Edema, weight gain, and elevated blood pressure

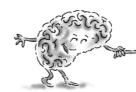

Central nervous system
- Headache
- Drowsiness
- Irritability
- Confusion
- Peripheral neuropathy
- Seizures
- Coma

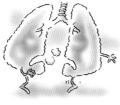

GI system
- Anorexia
- Nausea and vomiting
- Diarrhea or constipation
- Stomatitis
- Bleeding
- Hematemesis
- Dry mucous membranes
- Uremic breath

Respiratory system
- Pulmonary edema
- Kussmaul's respirations

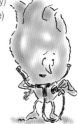

Integumentary system
- Dry skin
- Pruritus
- Pallor
- Purpura

Cardiovascular system
- Hypotension (early)
- Hypertension (late)
- Arrhythmias
- Fluid overload
- Heart failure
- Systemic edema
- Anemia
- Altered clotting mechanisms

Diuretic phase

- Slow increase in BUN and creatinine levels

▼

- Hypovolemia and weight loss

▼

- Decreased potassium, sodium, and water levels

▼

- Death if untreated

Recovery phase

- Normal BUN and creatinine levels with urine output between 1 and 2 L/day

Acute tubular necrosis

ATN causes 75% of all cases of acute renal failure.

Acute tubular necrosis (ATN), also called *acute tubulointerstitial nephritis*, destroys the tubular segment of the nephron, causing uremia (excess accumulation of protein metabolism by-products in blood) and renal failure.

How it happens

ATN results from ischemic or nephrotoxic injury, most commonly in debilitated patients, such as the critically ill and those who have undergone extensive surgery.

In ischemic injury, disruption of blood flow to the kidneys may result from circulatory collapse, severe hypotension, trauma, hemorrhage, dehydration, cardiogenic or septic shock, surgery, anesthetics, or reactions to transfusions. Ischemic ATN can damage the epithelial and basement membranes and cause lesions in the renal interstitium and is, therefore, irreversible.

Nephrotoxic injury may result from ingestion of certain chemical agents (such as contrast media administered during radiologic procedures), administration of antibiotics (aminoglycosides), or a hypersensitive reaction of the kidneys. Because nephrotoxic ATN doesn't damage the basement membrane of the nephron, it's potentially reversible.

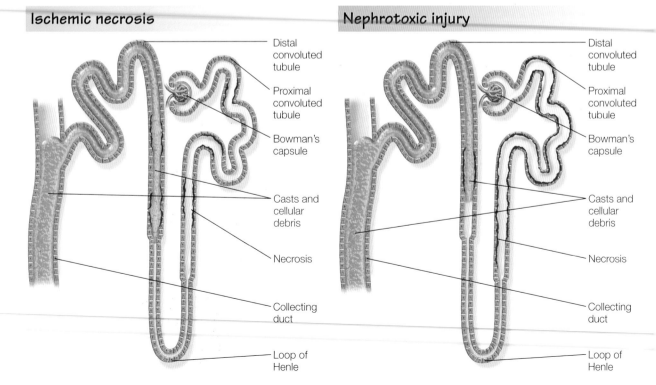

Ischemic necrosis

- Distal convoluted tubule
- Proximal convoluted tubule
- Bowman's capsule
- Casts and cellular debris
- Necrosis
- Collecting duct
- Loop of Henle

Nephrotoxic injury

- Distal convoluted tubule
- Proximal convoluted tubule
- Bowman's capsule
- Casts and cellular debris
- Necrosis
- Collecting duct
- Loop of Henle

What to look for

- Decreased urine output
- Hyperkalemia
- Uremic syndrome with oliguria (or, rarely, anuria) and confusion, which may progress to uremic coma
- Dry mucous membranes and skin
- Central nervous system signs and symptoms, such as lethargy, twitching, and seizures

ATN is usually difficult to recognize in its early stages because effects of the critically ill patient's primary disease may mask ATN's symptoms.

Pathogenesis of acute tubular necrosis

Necrosis and sloughing of epithelial cells result in the formation of casts, which causes obstruction and an increase in the intraluminal pressure, reducing the glomerular filtration rate. Vasoconstriction of the afferent arteriole, caused by tubuloglomerular feedback, results in decreased glomerular capillary filtration pressure. Injury to the tubule results and the increased intraluminal pressure causes fluid to leak back from the lumen into the interstitium.

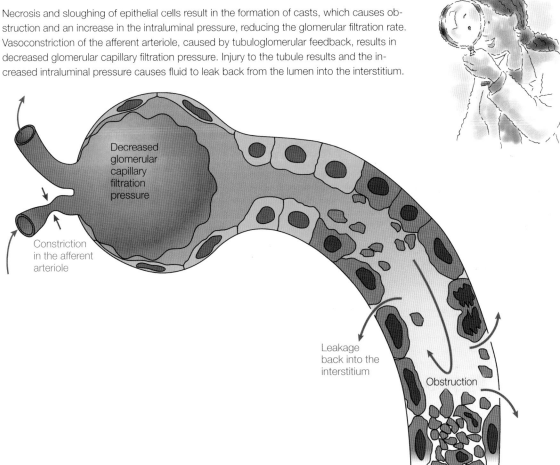

Decreased glomerular capillary filtration pressure

Constriction in the afferent arteriole

Leakage back into the interstitium

Obstruction

Glomerulonephritis

Glomerulonephritis is a bilateral inflammation of the glomeruli that commonly follows a streptococcal infection.

How it happens

In nearly all types of glomerulonephritis, the epithelial layer of the glomerular membrane is disturbed.

Acute poststreptococcal glomerulonephritis results from an immune response that occurs in the glomerulus. Glomerular injury occurs as a result of the inflammatory process.

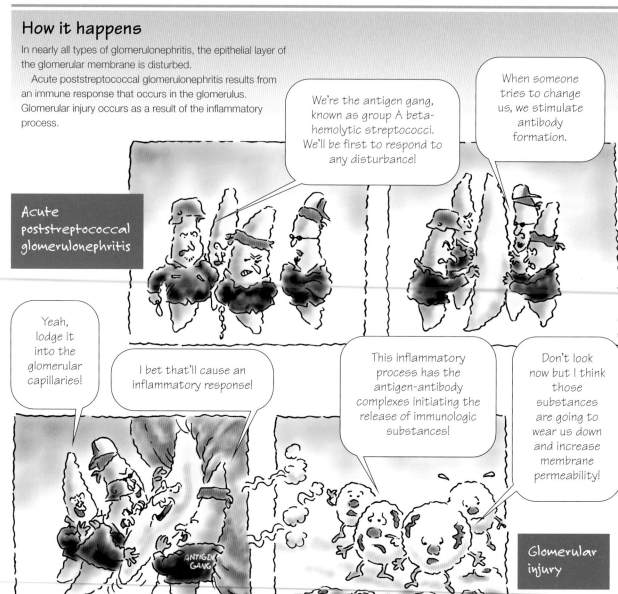

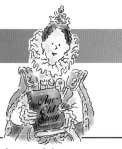

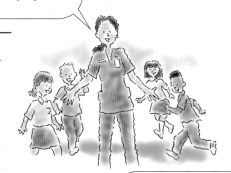

Acute glomerulonephritis is most common in boys ages 3 to 7 but it can occur at any age.

Age-old story

Age and glomerulonephritis

In children, the characteristic features of glomerulonephritis are usually encephalopathy with seizures and local neurologic deficits.

An elderly patient with glomerulonephritis may report vague, nonspecific symptoms, such as nausea, malaise, and arthralgia.

Immune complex deposits on the glomerulus

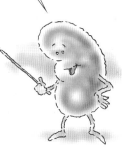

The severity of glomerular damage and renal insufficiency is related to the size, number, location, duration of exposure, and type of antigen-antibody complexes.

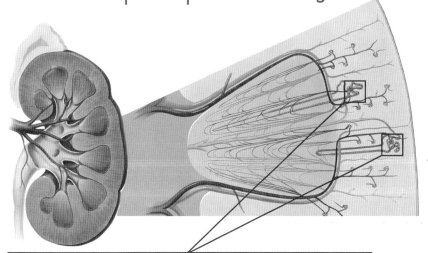

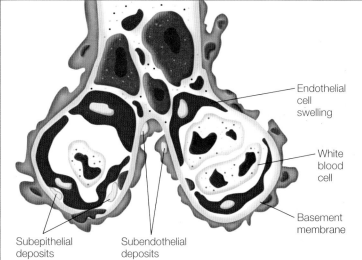

Endothelial cell swelling

White blood cell

Basement membrane

Subepithelial deposits

Subendothelial deposits

What to look for

- Decreased urination or oliguria
- Smoky or coffee-colored urine
- Shortness of breath
- Orthopnea
- Periorbital edema
- Mild to severe hypertension
- Bibasilar crackles on lung auscultation
- Nausea
- Malaise
- Arthralgia

Hydronephrosis

An abnormal dilation of the renal pelvis and the calyces of one or both kidneys, hydronephrosis is caused by an obstruction of urine flow in the genitourinary tract.

Almost any type of disease that results from obstruction of the urinary tract can result in hydronephrosis.

How it happens

If the obstruction is in the urethra or bladder, hydronephrosis usually affects both kidneys. If the obstruction is in a ureter, it usually affects one kidney. Obstructions distal to the bladder cause the bladder to dilate and act as a buffer zone, delaying hydronephrosis. Total obstruction of urine flow with dilation of the collecting system ultimately causes complete atrophy of the cortex (the outer portion of the kidney) and cessation of glomerular filtration.

Renal damage in hydronephrosis

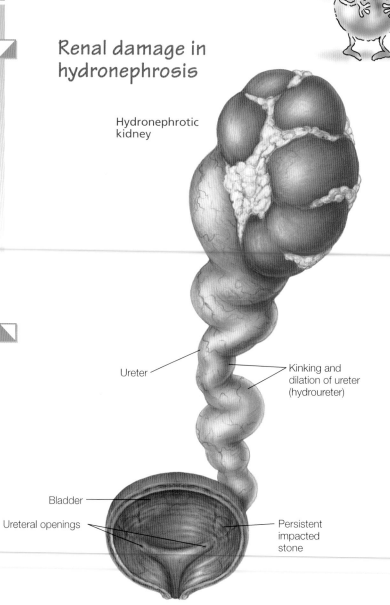

Hydronephrotic kidney

Ureter

Kinking and dilation of ureter (hydroureter)

Bladder

Ureteral openings

Persistent impacted stone

A closer look

This photograph shows dilation of the ureters, renal pelvises, and renal calyces from bilateral urinary tract obstruction.

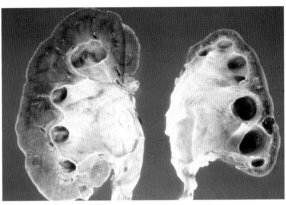

Cross section of hydronephrotic kidney

Dilated calyces

Atrophied parenchyma and tubules

Atrophied papilla

Dilated pelvis

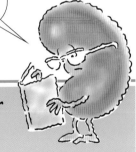

Signs and symptoms of hydronephrosis depend on the cause of the obstruction.

What to look for

Mild

- No symptoms
- Mild pain
- Slightly decreased urine flow

Severe

- Severe, colicky renal pain or dull flank pain
- Hematuria
- Pyuria
- Dysuria
- Alternating polyuria and oliguria, and complete anuria

General

- Nausea and vomiting
- Abdominal fullness
- Dribbling
- Urinary hesitancy

Polycystic kidney disease

Polycystic kidney disease is an inherited disorder characterized by multiple, bilateral, grapelike clusters of fluid-filled cysts that enlarge the kidneys, compressing and eventually replacing functioning renal tissue. The disease affects males and females equally and appears in three distinct forms.

Autosomal dominant polycystic kidney disease (ADPKD) is the most common type and accounts for about 10% of all cases of end-stage renal disease in the United States.

Another inherited form is called *autosomal recessive PKD*. It's a rare form that can exhibit symptoms when a fetus is still in the womb.

Acquired cystic kidney disease is the third form. This form isn't inherited and tends to occur in the later stages of life. It's associated with long-term kidney problems, especially kidney failure, and is prevalent in patients who have been receiving dialysis for a long period of time.

How it happens

Multiple spherical cysts, a few millimeters to centimeters in diameter and containing straw-colored or hemorrhagic fluid, cause grossly enlarged kidneys. The cysts are distributed evenly throughout the cortex and medulla. Hyperplastic polyps and renal adenomas are common. Renal parenchyma may have varying degrees of tubular atrophy, interstitial fibrosis, and nephrosclerosis. The cysts cause elongation of the renal pelvis, flattening of the calyces, and indentations in the kidney. Intracranial aneurysms, colonic diverticula, and mitral valve prolapse also occur.

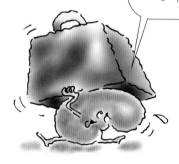

In most cases, progressive compression of kidney structures by the enlarging mass causes renal failure about 10 years after symptoms appear.

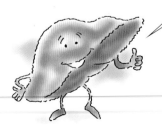

With polycystic kidney disease, I won't look this healthy for long. Cysts can develop on the liver, spleen, pancreas, and ovaries.

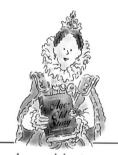

Age-old story

Age and polycystic kidney disease

Renal deterioration is more gradual in adults than infants. However, in both age-groups, the disease progresses relentlessly to fatal uremia.

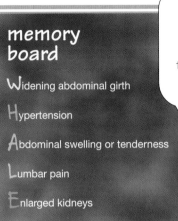

memory board

Widening abdominal girth

Hypertension

Abdominal swelling or tenderness

Lumbar pain

Enlarged kidneys

To remember the signs and symptoms of polycystic kidney disease, think about things that are enlarged, such as a WHALE!

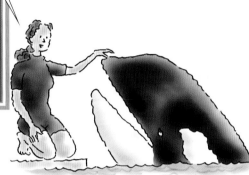

What to look for

- Hypertension
- Lumbar pain
- Widening abdominal girth
- Swollen or tender abdomen
- Grossly enlarged kidneys on palpation

Polycystic kidney

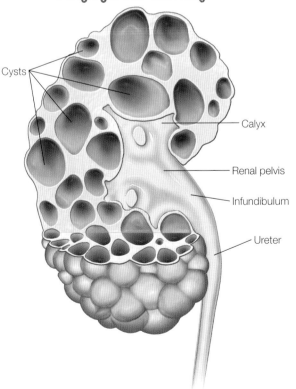

Cysts

Calyx

Renal pelvis

Infundibulum

Ureter

Adult polycystic disease

This photograph shows the enlarged, polycystic kidney of an adult (whole kidney on the left; cross-section on the right). Note that cysts have taken the place of almost all of the parenchyma.

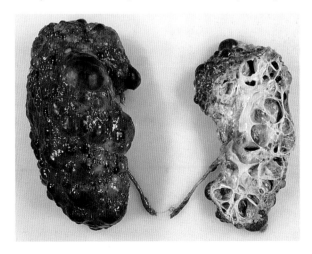

Pyelonephritis

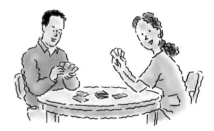

Chances are, I'll get pyelonephritis before he does!

Acute pyelonephritis, also known as *acute infective tubulointerstitial nephritis,* is a sudden inflammation caused by bacteria that primarily affects the interstitial area and the renal pelvis or, less commonly, the renal tubules. It's one of the most common renal diseases and may affect one or both kidneys. With treatment and continued follow-up care, the prognosis is good, and extensive permanent damage is rare.

Pyelonephritis is more common in females, probably because of the shorter female urethra and the proximity of the urinary meatus to the vagina and the rectum. Both conditions allow bacteria to reach the bladder more easily. In males, pyelonephritis may occur due to a lack of the antibacterial prostatic secretions normally produced in males.

How it happens

Typically, the infection spreads from the bladder to the ureters, then to the kidneys, as in vesicoureteral reflux. Vesicoureteral reflux may result from congenital weakness at the junction of the ureter and the bladder. Bacteria refluxed to intrarenal tissues may create colonies of infection within 24 to 48 hours. Infection may also result from instrumentation (such as catheterization, cystoscopy, or urologic surgery), from a hematogenic infection (as in septicemia or endocarditis) or, possibly, from lymphatic infection.

Pyelonephritis may also result from an inability to empty the bladder (for example, in patients with neurogenic bladder), urinary stasis, or urinary obstruction due to tumors, strictures, or benign prostatic hyperplasia.

Phases of pyelonephritis

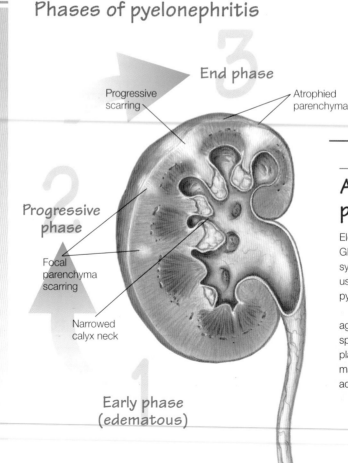

End phase

Progressive scarring

Atrophied parenchyma

Progressive phase

Focal parenchyma scarring

Narrowed calyx neck

Early phase (edematous)

Age-old story

Age and pyelonephritis

Elderly patients may exhibit GI or pulmonary signs and symptoms rather than the usual febrile responses to pyelonephritis.

In children younger than age 2, fever, vomiting, nonspecific abdominal complaints, and failure to thrive may be the only signs of acute pyelonephritis.

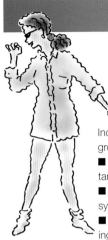

Risk factors for pyelonephritis

Incidence of pyelonephritis increases with age and is higher in the following groups:

■ *Sexually active women* — Intercourse increases the risk of bacterial contamination.

■ *Pregnant women* — About 5% develop bacteriuria that produces no symptoms; if untreated, about 40% develop pyelonephritis.

■ *People with diabetes* — Neurogenic bladder causes incomplete emptying and urinary stasis; glycosuria may support bacterial growth in the urine.

■ *People with other renal diseases* — Compromised renal function aggravates susceptibility.

What to look for

■ Urinary urgency and frequency, burning during urination, dysuria, nocturia, and hematuria

■ Cloudy urine that has an ammonia-like or fishy odor

■ Temperature of 102° F (38.9° C) or higher, shaking chills, nausea and vomiting, flank pain, anorexia, and general fatigue

A look at chronic pyelonephritis

These photographs show the effects of chronic pyelonephritis on the kidneys. In the first photo, you can see many reddish areas that indicate scarring. In the second photo, you can see severe dilation of the calyces as well as atrophy and scarring of the cortex.

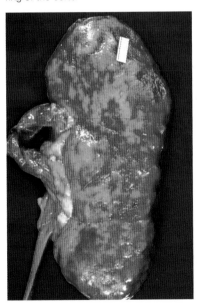
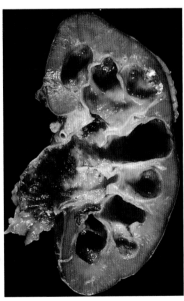

Renal calculi

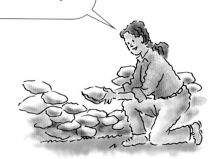

Some say good fences make good neighbors, but this many stones spells trouble for kidneys!

Also called *nephrolithiasis*, renal calculi (stones) can form anywhere in the urinary tract, although they most commonly develop in the renal pelves or calyces. They may vary in size and may be solitary or multiple.

The major types of renal calculi are calcium oxalate and calcium phosphate, accounting for 75% to 80% of calculi. Struvite (magnesium, ammonium, and phosphate) accounts for 15%; uric acid, 7%.

How it happens

Calculi form when substances that are normally dissolved in the urine, such as calcium oxalate and calcium phosphate, precipitate. Dehydration may lead to renal calculi as calculus-forming substances concentrate in urine.

Finish

Calculi may occur in the papillae, renal tubules, calyces, renal pelves, ureter, or bladder. Many calculi are less than 5 mm in diameter and are usually passed in the urine.

Staghorn calculi can continue to grow in the pelvis and extend to the calyces, forming a branching calculus and, ultimately, resulting in renal failure if not surgically removed.

Calculi may be composed of different substances, and the pH of the urine affects the solubility of many calculus-forming substances.

Hop along with me and see how it all happens!

A crystal evolves in the presence of calculus-forming substances (calcium oxalate, calcium carbonate, magnesium, ammonium, phosphate, or uric acid) and becomes trapped in the urinary tract, where it attracts other crystals to form a calculus.

A high urine saturation of these substances encourages crystal formation and results in calculus growth.

Calculi form around a nucleus in the appropriate environment.

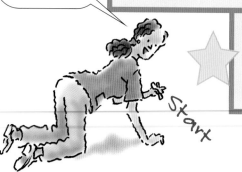

Start

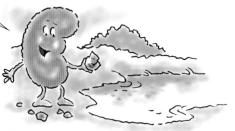

Types of renal calculi

Uric acid stones

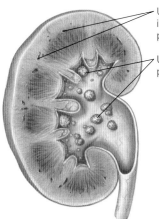

Urate deposits in renal parenchyma

Urate stones in pelvis

Ammoniomagnesium phosphate (struvite) stones

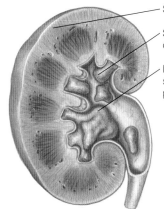

Slight renal edema

Stone forming in calyx

Large "staghorn" stone in renal pelvis

A look at staghorn calculi

This photo shows a kidney with hydronephrosis and staghorn calculi, which are casts of the dilated calyces.

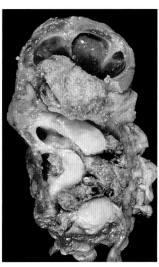

Calcium stones

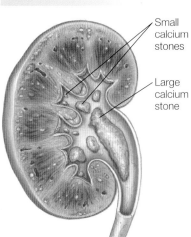

Small calcium stones

Large calcium stone

What to look for

■ Pain resulting from obstruction (possibly mild to severe deep flank pain or tenderness; or abrupt, severe, colicky flank pain)
■ Nausea and vomiting
■ Fever and chills (from infection)
■ Hematuria (when calculi abrade a ureter)
■ Urinary hesitancy and dysuria (due to obstruction)
■ Abdominal distention
■ Anuria (from bilateral obstruction or obstruction of a patient's only kidney)

Renovascular hypertension

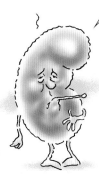

I can just feel the renin risin'. Nobody knows the trouble I've seen...

Renovascular hypertension occurs when systemic blood pressure increases due to intrarenal atherosclerosis or stenosis of the major renal arteries or their branches. This narrowing (sclerosis) may be partial or complete, and the resulting blood pressure elevation may be benign or malignant. Renovascular hypertension is the most common type of secondary hypertension.

How it happens

The kidneys normally play a key role in maintaining blood pressure and volume by vasoconstriction and regulation of sodium and fluid levels. In renovascular hypertension, these regulatory mechanisms fail.

1 Certain conditions, such as renal artery stenosis and tumors, reduce blood flow to the kidneys. This reduced flow causes juxtaglomerular cells to continuously secrete renin—an enzyme that converts angiotensinogen (a plasma protein) to angiotensin I.

In this stage, be alert for flank pain, systolic bruit in the epigastric vein over the upper abdomen, reduced urine output, and an elevated renin level.

2 In the liver, renin and angiotensinogen combine to form angiotensin I, which converts to angiotensin II in the lungs. This potent vasoconstrictor heightens peripheral resistance and blood pressure.

Check for headache, nausea, anorexia, an elevated renin level, and hypertension.

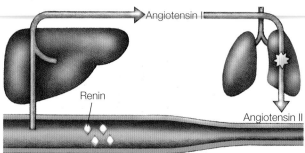

Angiotensin I

Renin

Angiotensin II

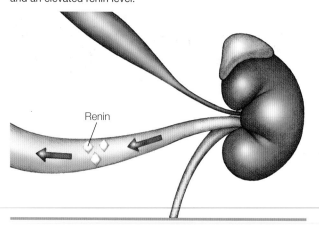

Renin

Angiotensin II acts directly on the kidneys, causing them to reabsorb sodium and water.

Assess for hypertension, diminished urine output, albuminuria, hypokalemia, and hypernatremia.

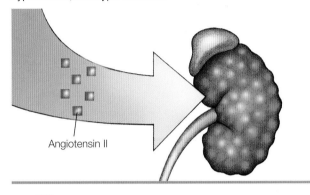

Angiotensin II

Angiotensin II stimulates the adrenal cortex to secrete aldosterone and also causes the kidneys to retain sodium and water, elevating blood volume and pressure.

Expect worsening symptoms.

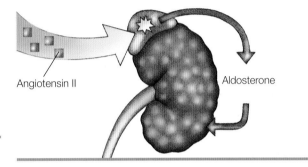

Angiotensin II   Aldosterone

Intermittent pressure diuresis causes excretion of sodium and water, reduced blood volume, and decreasing cardiac output.

Check for blood pressure that increases slowly, drops (but not as low as before), and then increases again. Headache, high urine specific gravity, hyponatremia, fatigue, and heart failure also occur.

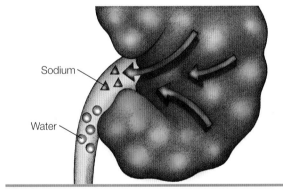

Sodium

Water

A high aldosterone level causes further sodium retention, but it can't curtail renin secretion. Excessive aldosterone and angiotensin II can damage renal tissue, leading to renal failure.

Expect to find hypertension, pitting edema, anemia, decreased level of consciousness, and elevated blood urea nitrogen and serum creatinine levels.

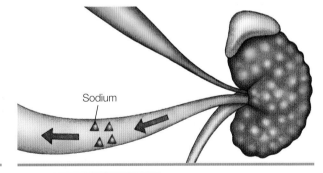

Sodium

What to look for

- ■ Flank pain
- ■ Systolic bruit over the epigastric vein in the upper abdomen
- ■ Reduced urine output
- ■ Headache
- ■ Nausea
- ■ Anorexia
- ■ Anxiety
- ■ Hypertension
- ■ Altered level of consciousness
- ■ Pitting edema

VISION QUEST

Able to label?

In the illustration, label the three classifications of acute renal disease.

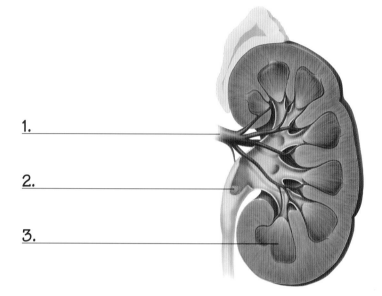

1. _____

2. _____

3. _____

Rebus riddle

Solve the riddle to discover the place where you'll find a renal disorder.

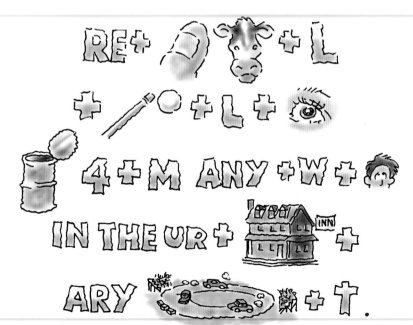

11
Integumentary disorders

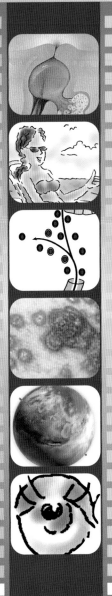

Make-up can be a lifesaver for movie stars when they need to hide those unsightly blemishes from the big screen. Other skin disorders need medical attention!

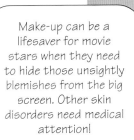

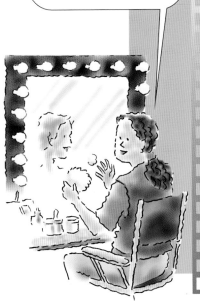

Acne

Acne is a chronic inflammatory disease of the sebaceous glands. It's usually associated with a high rate of sebum secretion and occurs on areas of the body that contain sebaceous glands, such as the face, neck, chest, back, and shoulders. There are two types of acne:

Inflammatory, in which the hair follicle is blocked by sebum, causing bacteria to grow and eventually rupture the follicle

Noninflammatory, in which the follicle doesn't rupture but remains dilated.

How it happens

1
Excessive sebum production

Androgens stimulate sebaceous gland growth and the production of sebum, which is secreted into dilated hair follicles that contain bacteria.

2
Increased shedding of epithelial cells

The bacteria, usually *Propionibacterium acne* and *Staphylococcus epidermidis,* are normal skin flora that secrete the enzyme lipase. This enzyme interacts with sebum to produce free fatty acids, which provoke inflammation.

Epithelial cells   Sebaceous follicle

Blocked follicle

Epidermis

Dermis

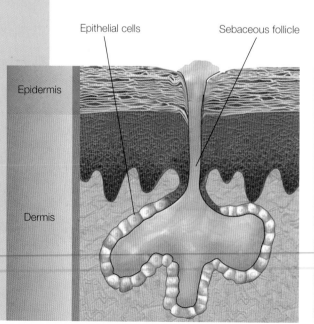

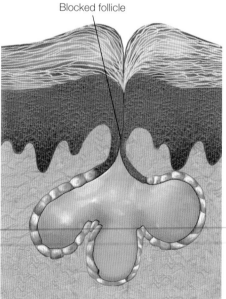

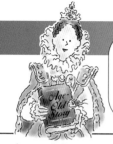

Age-old story

Age and acne

Acne occurs in both males and females. Acne vulgaris develops in 80% to 90% of adolescents or young adults, primarily between ages 15 and 18.

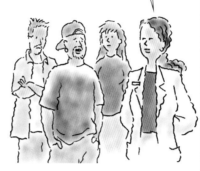

> Although lesions can appear as early as age 8, acne primarily affects adolescents. Sorry, guys!

Adolescent facial acne

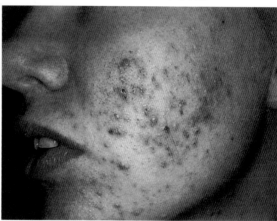

3

Inflammatory response in follicle

Hair follicles also produce more keratin, which joins with the sebum to form a plug in the dilated follicle.

Ruptured follicle

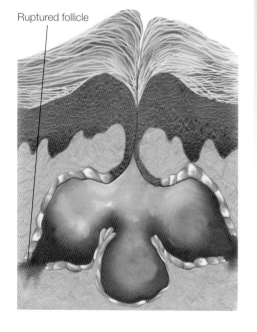

What to look for

The acne plug may appear as:
- a closed comedo, or whitehead (may be protruding from the follicle and covered by the epidermis)
- an open comedo, or blackhead (protruding from the follicle and not covered by the epidermis; melanin or pigment of the follicle causes the black color)
- inflammation
- acne pustules, papules or, in severe forms, acne cysts or abscesses.

Comedones of acne

Closed comedo (whitehead)

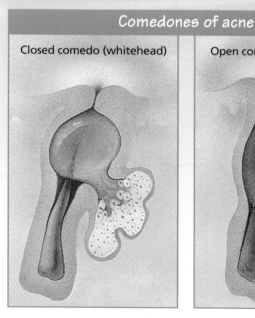

Open comedo (blackhead)

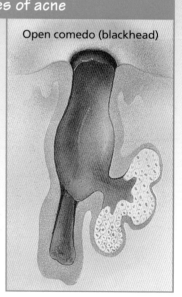

Burns

I'd better be careful or I'll get a superficial partial-thickness burn...

Burns are classified as superficial partial-thickness (first-degree), deep partial-thickness (second-degree), full-thickness (third-degree), and full-thickness involving muscle, bone, and interstitial tissue (fourth-degree).

How it happens

The injuring agent denatures cellular proteins. Some cells die because of traumatic or ischemic necrosis. Loss of collagen cross-linking also occurs with denaturation, creating abnormal osmotic and hydrostatic pressure gradients, which cause the movement of intravascular fluid into interstitial spaces. Cellular injury triggers the release of mediators of inflammation, contributing to local and, in the case of major burns, systemic increases in capillary permeability. Specific pathophysiologic events depend on the burn's cause and classification.

Superficial partial-thickness burns

A superficial partial-thickness burn causes localized injury or destruction to the epidermis only by direct (such as chemical spill) or indirect (such as sunlight) contact. The barrier function of the skin remains intact.

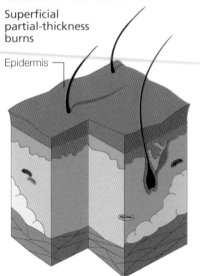

Superficial partial-thickness burns

Epidermis

Deep partial-thickness burns

Deep partial-thickness burns involve destruction to the epidermis and some dermis. Thin-walled, fluid-filled blisters develop within a few minutes of the injury along with mild to

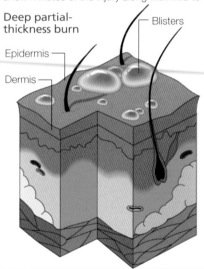

Deep partial-thickness burn

Epidermis

Dermis

Blisters

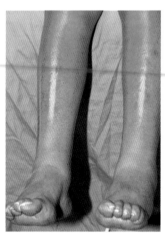

Superficial thermal burn (sunburn)

What to look for

Superficial partial-thickness burn

- Localized pain and erythema, usually without blisters in the first 24 hours, caused by injury from direct or indirect contact with a burn source
- Chills, headache, localized edema, and nausea and vomiting (with more severe superficial partial-thickness burn)
- Thin-walled, fluid-filled blisters appearing within minutes of the injury, with mild to moderate edema and pain (with deep partial-thickness burn)
- White, waxy appearance to damaged area (deep partial-thickness burn)

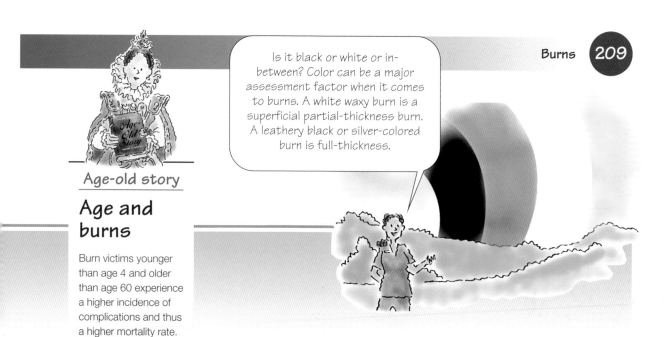

Age and burns

Burn victims younger than age 4 and older than age 60 experience a higher incidence of complications and thus a higher mortality rate.

moderate edema and pain. As these blisters break, the nerve endings become exposed to the air. Pain and tactile responses remain intact so subsequent treatments are painful. The barrier function of the skin is lost.

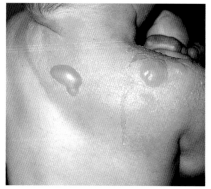

Deep partial-thickness burn (sunburn)

Full-thickness burns

A major full-thickness burn affects every body system and organ. A full-thickness burn extends through the epidermis and dermis and into the subcutaneous tissue layer. If the burn is fourth-degree, muscle, bone, and interstitial tissues would also be involved. Within hours, fluids and protein shift from capillary to interstitial spaces, causing edema. The immediate immunologic response to the burn injury makes burn wound sepsis a potential threat. Lastly, an increase in calorie demand after the burn injury increases metabolic rate.

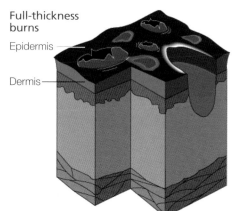

Full-thickness burns

Epidermis
Dermis

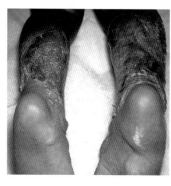

Full-thickness burns to the legs

Full-thickness burn

■ White, brown, or black leathery tissue and visible thrombosed vessels due to destruction of skin elasticity (the dorsum of the hand is the most common site of thrombosed veins), without blisters
■ Silver-colored, raised area, usually at the site of electrical contact (with electrical burn)
■ Singed nasal hairs, mucosal burns, voice changes, coughing, wheezing, soot in mouth or nose, and darkened sputum (with smoke inhalation and pulmonary damage).

Cellulitis

Cellulitis is an infection of the dermis or subcutaneous layer of the skin. It may follow damage to the skin, such as a bite or wound. As the cellulitis spreads, fever, erythema, and lymphangitis may occur.

If cellulitis is treated in a timely manner, the prognosis is usually good.

Age-old story

Age and cellulitis

Cellulitis of the lower extremity is more likely to develop into thrombophlebitis in an elderly patient.

How it happens

As the offending organism invades the compromised area, it overwhelms the defensive cells (neutrophils, eosinophils, basophils, and mast cells) that break down the cellular components, which normally contain and localize the inflammation. As cellulitis progresses, the organism invades tissue around the initial wound site.

Phases of acute inflammatory response

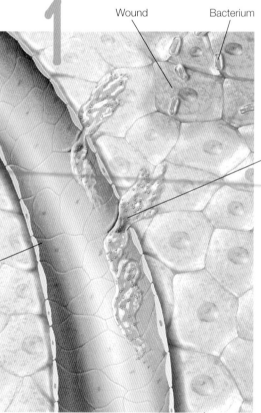

Wound

Bacterium

Increased blood flow carrying plasma proteins and fluid to the injured tissue

Blood vessel

I've got you under my skin— and I want you out!

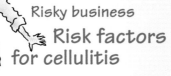

Risky business

Risk factors for cellulitis

- Diabetes
- Immunodeficiency
- Impaired circulation
- Neuropathy

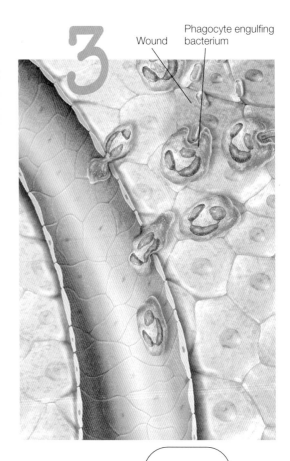

Wound

Phagocyte engulfing bacterium

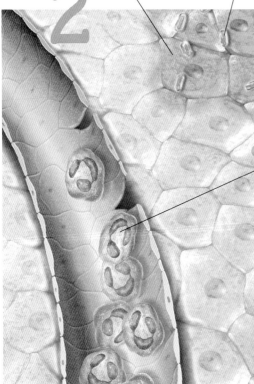

Wound

Bacterium

Movement of defensive white blood cells to injured tissue

Recognizing cellulitis

The classic signs of cellulitis are erythema and edema surrounding the initial wound. The tissue is warm to the touch.

Now that's hot!

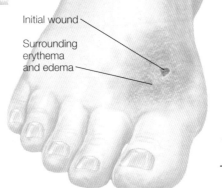

Initial wound

Surrounding erythema and edema

What to look for

- Erythema and edema
- Pain and warmth at the site and, possibly, surrounding area
- Fever

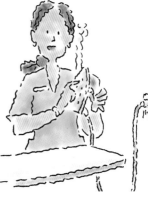

Contact dermatitis

Contact dermatitis commonly appears as a sharply demarcated inflammation of the skin resulting from contact with an irritating chemical or atopic allergen (a substance producing an allergic reaction in the skin). It can also appear as an irritation of the skin resulting from contact with concentrated substances to which the skin is sensitive, such as perfumes, soaps, chemicals, or metals and alloys (for instance, the nickel used in jewelry).

Your patients don't have to hide their dermatitis from the world! They just have to be careful of their sensitive skin!

How it happens

1 Hapten of toxicodendron origin

2 Hapten-carrier complex formed at Langerhans' cell membrane. Requires 1 hour.

Langerhans' cell

3 Processed antigen presented to the T cells. Processing, presentation, and sensitization takes 24 hours.

Hapten-carrier complex

T cells

Sensitized T cells

4 Sensitized T cells enter a lymphatic vessel.

Lymphatic vessel

5 Sensitized T cells transported to regional lymph nodes, where T-cell hyperplasia is induced.

What to look for

■ Erythema and small vesicles that ooze, scale, and itch (due to mild irritants and allergens)
■ Blisters and ulcerations (due to strong irritants)
■ Clearly defined lesions, with straight lines following points of contact (classic allergic response)
■ Marked erythema, blistering, and edema of affected areas (severe allergic reaction)

Contact dermatitis from nickel of watch on skin

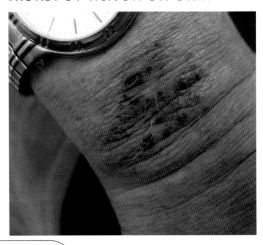

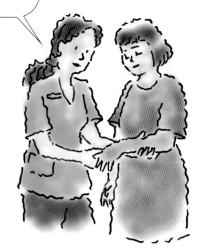

Looks like you've been scratching again!

6

Sensitized T cells return to dermis and epidermis.

Lymph node

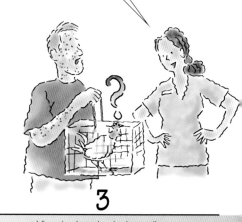

I said, "It looks like you have chickenpox," not "a chicken in a box."

Herpes zoster

Herpes zoster, also called *shingles*, is an acute inflammation caused by infection with human herpesvirus 3 (varicella-zoster virus [VZV], or chickenpox virus). It usually occurs in adults and produces localized vesicular skin lesions and severe neuralgic pain in peripheral areas. Complete recovery is common, but scarring may occur as well as vision impairment (with corneal damage) or persistent neuralgia.

1	**2**	**3**
Varicella zoster virus (chickenpox)	Non-immune individual (usually a child)	Virus in dorsal spinal ganglion (latent phase)

How it happens

An individual (usually a child) develops chickenpox through droplet transmission or inhalation of the varicella or chickenpox virus. The virus initially causes a "silent" infection of the nasopharynx. This infection progresses to viremia, seeding of fixed macrophages, and dissemination of VZV to the skin (the rash seen in chickenpox).

After the initial infection, the virus lays dormant in the dorsal spinal ganglion, where it remains for many years. The virus is reactivated, probably because of decreased cellular immunity, and spreads from ganglia along the sensory nerves to the peripheral nerves of sensory dermatomes, causing shingles.

Dormant?! I can't believe there's anything dormant in this little guy.

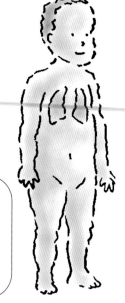

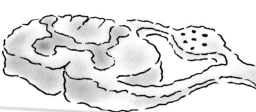

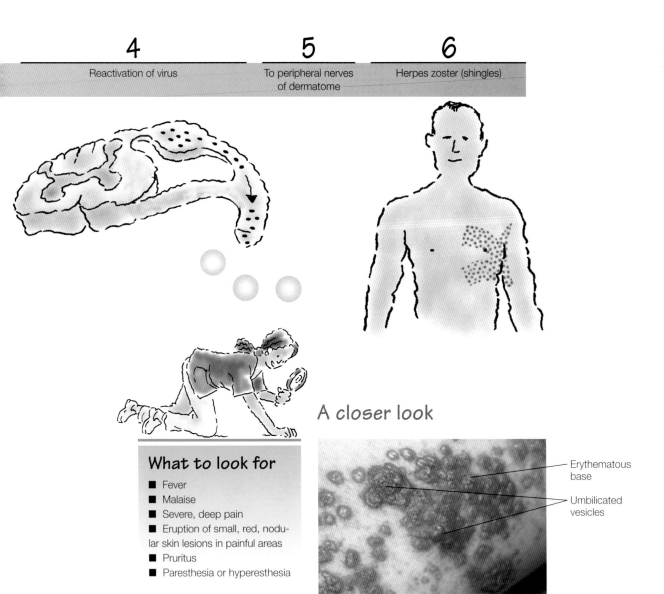

4

Reactivation of virus

5

To peripheral nerves
of dermatome

6

Herpes zoster (shingles)

What to look for

- Fever
- Malaise
- Severe, deep pain
- Eruption of small, red, nodular skin lesions in painful areas
- Pruritus
- Paresthesia or hyperesthesia

A closer look

Erythematous base

Umbilicated vesicles

Malignant melanoma

Malignant melanoma is the most lethal skin cancer. It accounts for 1% to 2% of all malignant tumors and it's slightly more common in women than men.

How it happens

Malignant melanoma arises from melanocytes (cells that synthesize the pigment melanin). In addition to the skin, melanocytes are also found in the meninges, alimentary canal, respiratory tract, and lymph nodes.

Melanoma spreads through the lymphatic and vascular systems and metastasizes to the regional lymph nodes, skin, liver, lungs, and central nervous system. In most patients, superficial lesions are curable, but deeper lesions are more likely to metastasize.

Up to 70% of malignant melanomas arise from a preexisting nevus (circumscribed malformation of the skin) or mole.

Understanding skin cancer

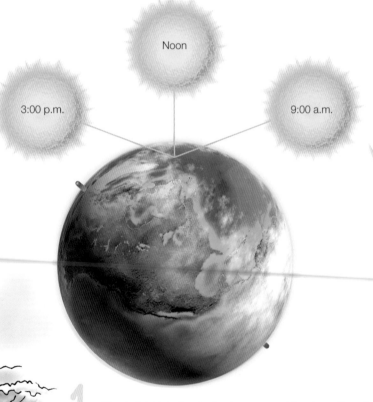

Noon

3:00 p.m.

9:00 a.m.

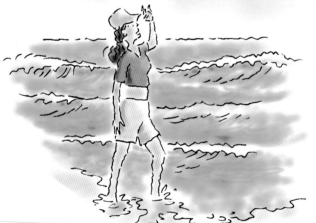

1 Due to the changing angle of our sun and the absorption of solar radiation by our atmosphere, the intensity of ultraviolet (UV) radiation striking the surface of the earth at noon is twice as strong as radiation striking the earth in the early morning and late afternoon.

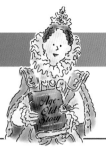

Age and malignant melanoma

Malignant melanoma is unusual in children, and occurs most commonly between ages 40 and 50. However, the incidence in younger age-groups is increasing because of increased sun exposure or, possibly, a decrease in the ozone layer.

2 UVA and UVB absorption by deoxyribonucleic acid (DNA) and other structures inside the nuclei of skin cells leads to cellular and molecular damage (sunburn), including pain, inflammation, swelling, and loss of function.

3 Incomplete or incorrect repair of UV radiation–induced DNA damage is largely responsible for the growth of precancerous cells and malignant cells.

Nucleus

DNA

Arteriole

Keratinocyte (can become squamous cell carcinoma)

Melanocyte (can become melanoma)

Basal cell (can become basal cell carcinoma)

1 Golgi apparatus (produces melanosomes)

2 Melanosomes (develop into granules)

3 Melanin granules (store melanin pigment for transport to keratinocytes)

Melanocytes located in the basal layer of the epidermis produce melanin, a pigment that's responsible for the various skin colors.

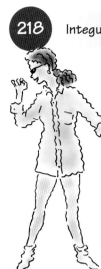

Risky business
Risk factors for melanoma

- Excessive exposure to sunlight
- Increased nevi
- Tendency to freckle from the sun
- Hormonal factors such as pregnancy
- A family history or past history of melanoma
- Red hair, fair skin, blue eyes, susceptibility to sunburn, and Celtic or Scandinavian ancestry (Melanoma is rare in blacks.)

Did you say red hair, fair skin, and blue eyes? Drats! Bring me the sunscreen!

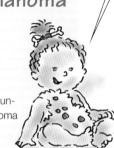

What to look for
Changes to a preexisting skin lesion or nevus

- Enlarges
- Changes color
- Becomes inflamed or sore
- Itches
- Ulcerates
- Bleeds
- Changes texture
- Shows signs of surrounding pigment regression

A closer look

Malignant melanoma can arise on normal skin or from an existing mole. If not treated promptly, it can spread to other areas of skin, lymph nodes, or internal organs.

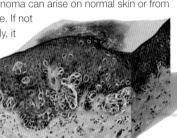

Common sites for malignant melanoma are the head and neck in men and the legs in women. So wear that sunblock or put on a hat and pants!

Memory board
ABCDEs of malignant melanoma

Asymmetrical lesion

Border irregular

Color of lesion varies with shades of tan, brown, or black and, possibly, red, blue, or white

Diameter greater than 6 mm

Elevated or enlarging lesion

Just as I suspected. Lots of clues here that lead me straight to malignant melanoma.

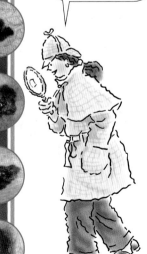

Pressure ulcers

Pressure ulcers, commonly called *pressure sores* or *bedsores*, are localized areas of cellular necrosis that occur most often in the skin and subcutaneous tissue over bony prominences. These ulcers may be superficial (caused by local skin irritation with subsequent surface maceration) or deep (originating in underlying tissue). Deep lesions commonly remain undetected until they penetrate the skin, but by then they have usually caused subcutaneous damage.

Most pressure ulcers develop over five body locations:

1 Sacral area   **2** Lateral malleolus   **3** Ischial tuberosity   **4** Greater trochanter   **5** Heel

Collectively, these areas account for 95% of all pressure ulcer sites. Patients who have contractures are at an increased risk for developing pressure ulcers because of the added pressure on the tissue and the alignment of the bones.

Pressure ulcers are categorized as stage I, stage II, stage III, or stage IV.

memory board

Sacral area

Lateral malleolus

Ischial tuberosity

Greater trochanter

Heel

Here's a SLIGH way to remember the five body locations where pressure ulcers commonly develop.

How it happens

A pressure ulcer is caused by an injury to the skin and its underlying tissues. The pressure exerted on the area causes ischemia and hypoxemia to the affected tissues because of decreased blood flow to the site.

As the capillaries collapse, thrombosis occurs, which subsequently leads to tissue edema and then tissue necrosis.

Ischemia also adds to an accumulation of waste products at the site, which in turn leads to the production of toxins. The toxins further break down the tissue and eventually lead to the death of the cells.

When ischemia is in town, there's always an accumulation of waste products.

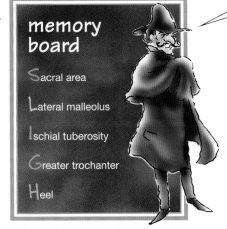

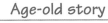

Age-old story

Age and pressure ulcers

Age plays a role in the incidence of pressure ulcers. Muscle is lost with aging, and skin elasticity decreases. Both of these factors increase the risk of developing pressure ulcers.

What to look for

Pressure ulcer staging

Stage I

A stage I pressure ulcer is an area of skin with observable pressure-related changes when compared to an adjacent area or to the same region on the other side of the body. Indicators include a change in one or more of these characteristics:

- skin temperature (warmth or coolness)
- tissue consistency (boggy or firm)
- sensation (pain or itching).

This ulcer presents clinically as a defined area of persistent redness in patients with light skin or persistent red, blue, or purple in patients with darker skin.

Stage II

A stage II pressure ulcer is a superficial partial-thickness wound that presents clinically as an abrasion, a blister, or a shallow crater involving the epidermis and dermis.

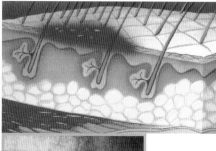

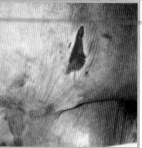

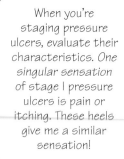

> When you're staging pressure ulcers, evaluate their characteristics. One singular sensation of stage I pressure ulcers is pain or itching. These heels give me a similar sensation!

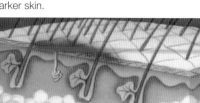

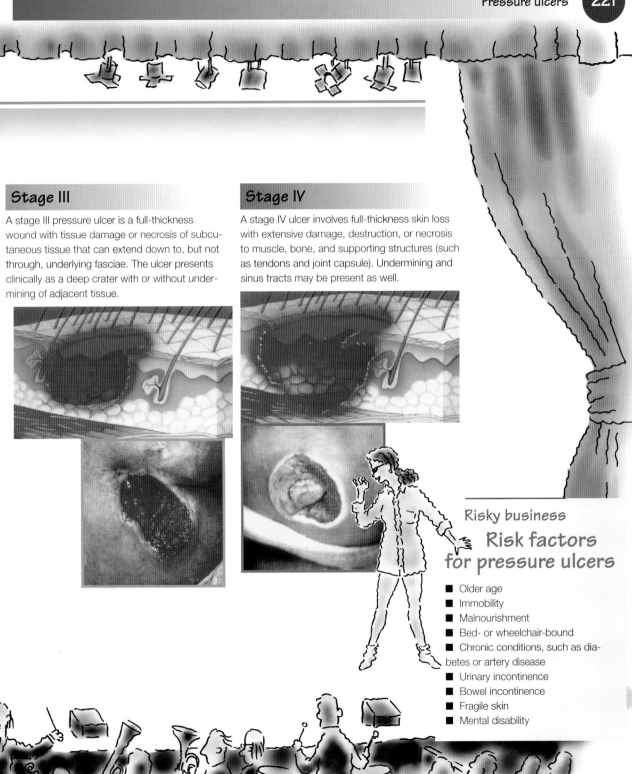

Stage III

A stage III pressure ulcer is a full-thickness wound with tissue damage or necrosis of subcutaneous tissue that can extend down to, but not through, underlying fasciae. The ulcer presents clinically as a deep crater with or without undermining of adjacent tissue.

Stage IV

A stage IV ulcer involves full-thickness skin loss with extensive damage, destruction, or necrosis to muscle, bone, and supporting structures (such as tendons and joint capsule). Undermining and sinus tracts may be present as well.

Risky business
Risk factors for pressure ulcers

- Older age
- Immobility
- Malnourishment
- Bed- or wheelchair-bound
- Chronic conditions, such as diabetes or artery disease
- Urinary incontinence
- Bowel incontinence
- Fragile skin
- Mental disability

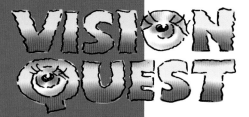

Show and tell

Identify the three types of burns in each illustration and indicate their characteristics.

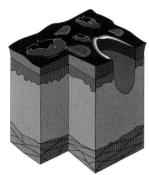
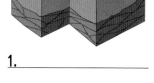
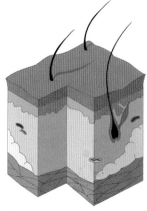
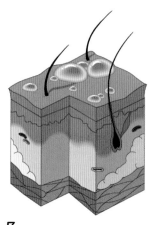

1._____
_____
_____
_____
_____
_____
_____

2._____
_____
_____
_____
_____
_____
_____

3._____
_____
_____
_____
_____
_____
_____

Matchmaker

Match the definitions with their corresponding disorders.

1. Most lethal skin cancer ____
2. Localized areas of cellular necrosis that are most common over bony prominences ____
3. Chronic inflammatory disease of the sebaceous glands ____
4. Inflammation or irritation of the skin due to contact with irritating chemical or atopic allergen ____
5. Infection of the dermis or subcutaneous layer of the skin ____
6. Acute inflammation caused by infection with herpesvirus ____

A. Cellulitis
B. Herpes zoster
C. Acne
D. Contact dermatitis
E. Malignant melanoma
F. Pressure ulcers

Answers: Show and tell 1. Full-thickness; extends through the epidermis and dermis and into the subcutaneous tissue layer 2. partial-thickness; causes localized injury or destruction to the epidermis only 3. deep partial-thickness; involves destruction to the epidermis and some dermis Matchmaker 1. E, 2. F, 3. C, 4. D, 5. A, 6. B.

12
Reproductive disorders

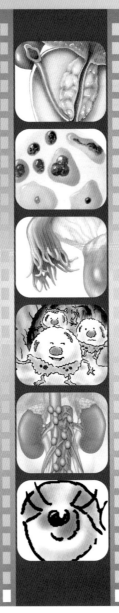

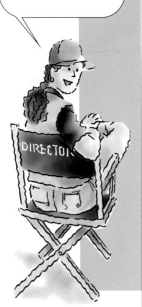

I've seen some great endings in my line of work, but finishing with the reproductive chapter? It's brilliant!

Benign prostatic hyperplasia

Although most men age 50 and older have some prostatic enlargement, in benign prostatic hyperplasia (BPH)—also known as *benign prostatic hypertrophy* or *nodular hyperplasia*—the prostate gland enlarges enough to compress the urethra and cause overt urinary obstruction.

How it happens

Regardless of the cause, BPH begins with nonmalig-nant changes in periurethral glandular tissue. The growth of the fibroadenomatous nodules (masses of fibrous glandular tissue) progresses to compress the remaining normal gland (nodular hy-perplasia). The hyperplastic tissue is mostly glandular, with some fibrous stroma and smooth muscle.

As the prostate enlarges, it may extend into the blad-der and obstruct urinary outflow by compressing or distorting the prostatic ure-thra. Periodic increases in sympathetic stimulation of the smooth muscle of the prostatic urethra and blad-der neck also occur. Pro-gressive bladder distention may cause a pouch to form in the bladder that retains urine when the rest of the bladder empties. This re-tained urine may lead to cal-culus formation or cystitis.

Prostatic enlargement

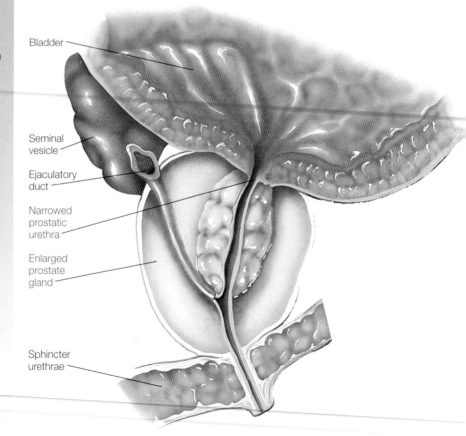

Bladder

Seminal vesicle

Ejaculatory duct

Narrowed prostatic urethra

Enlarged prostate gland

Sphincter urethrae

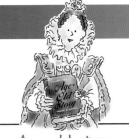

Age and BPH

BPH is common, affecting up to 50% of men age 50 and older, and 80% to 90% of men age 80 and older.

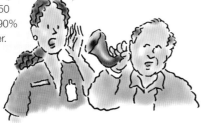

I said, "Have you had your prostate checked lately?"

Risk factors for BPH

- Age
- Family history of BPH

Nodular hyperplasia of the prostate

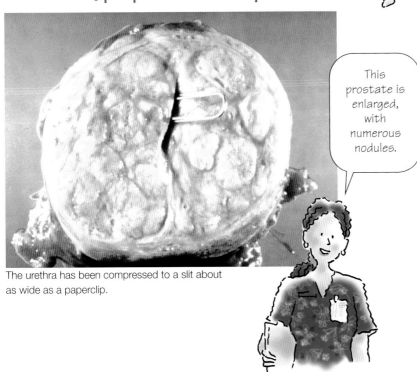

This prostate is enlarged, with numerous nodules.

The urethra has been compressed to a slit about as wide as a paperclip.

What to look for

Signs and symptoms of BPH depend on the extent of prostatic enlargement and the lobes affected. Characteristically, the condition starts with a group of symptoms known as *prostatism,* which are caused by enlargement, and include:

- reduced urine stream caliber and force
- urinary hesitancy
- difficulty starting micturition (resulting in straining, feeling of incomplete voiding, and an interrupted stream).

As the obstruction increases, it causes:

- frequent urination with nocturia
- sense of urgency
- dribbling
- urine retention
- incontinence
- possible hematuria.

Breast cancer

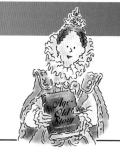

Breast cancer is the most common cancer in women. Breast cancer ranks second among cancer deaths in women, behind cancer of the lung and bronchus.

Age and breast cancer

Although the disease may develop any time after puberty, 70% of cases occur in women older than age 50.

How it happens

Slow-growing breast cancer spreads by way of the lymphatic system and the bloodstream, through the right side of the heart to the lungs, and eventually to the other breast, the chest wall, liver, bone, and brain.

Most breast cancers arise from the ductal epithelium. Tumors of the infiltrating ductal type don't enlarge dramatically, but metastasize early.

> Breast cancer occurs more frequently in the left breast than the right and more commonly in the outer upper quadrant.

Types of breast cancer

Ductal carcinoma in situ

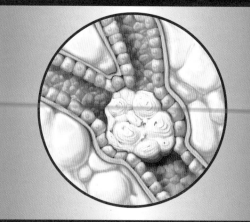

Infiltrating (invasive) ductal carcinoma

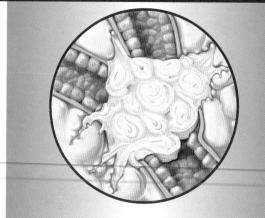

Classifying breast cancer

Breast cancer is classified by histologic appearance and location of the lesion:
- adenocarcinoma—arises from the epithelium
- intraductal—occurs within the ducts (including Paget's disease)
- infiltrating—appears in parenchymal tissue of the breast
- inflammatory (rare)—overlying skin becomes edematous, inflamed, and indurated; reflects rapid tumor growth
- lobular carcinoma in situ—involves glandular lobes
- medullary or circumscribed—appears as a large tumor, with rapid growth rate.

Staging of breast cancer

Stage I

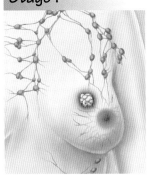

In stage I, the tumor is less than 2 cm in size; there are no axillary or other metastases.

Stage II

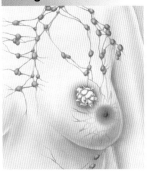

In stage II, the tumor is greater than 2 cm in size; there may be nonfixed axillary metastasis but it doesn't extend into other areas.

Stage III

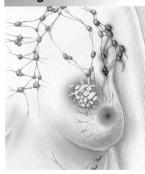

In stage III, the tumor is greater than 5 cm in size; there's fixed axillary but no other metastasis.

Stage IV

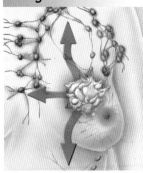

In stage IV, the tumor can be any size, supraclavicular or intraclavicular nodes are affected, and there's distant metastasis.

Risky business
Risk factors for breast cancer

Higher risk

- Family history of breast cancer, particularly first-degree relatives (mother or sister)
- Genetic mutations in BRCA-1 and BRCA-2 genes (suggest genetic predisposition)
- Long menses (menses beginning early or menopause beginning late)
- No history of pregnancy
- History of bilateral breast cancer
- History of endometrial or ovarian cancer
- Exposure to low-level ionizing radiation

Lower risk

- History of pregnancy before age 20
- History of multiple pregnancies
- Native American or Asian ethnicity

Genetic mutations are just one of the major risk factors for breast cancer. OK, everyone, let's see what we end up with when everyone does left foot blue.

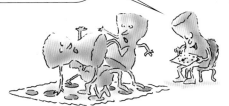

Carcinoma of the breast

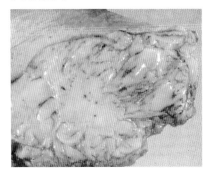

What to look for

- Thickening of the breast tissue
- Painless lump or mass in the breast
- Nipple retraction
- Scaly skin around the nipple
- Skin changes
- Erythema
- Clear, milky, or bloody discharge
- Edema in the arm, indicating advanced nodal involvement
- Cervical supraclavicular and axillary node lumps or enlargement

Cervical cancer

Cervical cancer is the third most common cancer of the female reproductive system and is classified as either invasive or microinvasive. Preinvasive disease, also known as *precancerous dysplasia, cervical intraepithelial carcinoma*, or *cervical cancer in situ*, is more frequent than invasive cancer and occurs more commonly in younger women.

How it happens

Preinvasive disease can range from mild cervical dysplasia (in which the lower third of the epithelium contains abnormal cells), to carcinoma in situ (in which the full thickness of epithelium contains abnormally proliferating cells).

In invasive carcinoma, cancer cells penetrate the basement membrane and can spread directly to adjacent pelvic structures or disseminate to distant sites by lymphatic routes.

A closer look

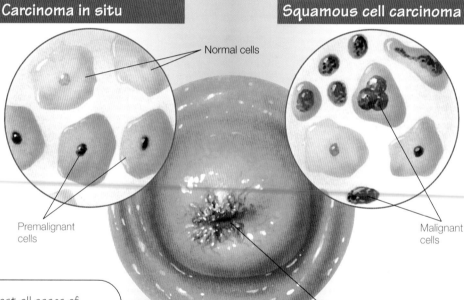

Carcinoma in situ

Squamous cell carcinoma

Normal cells

Premalignant cells

Malignant cells

Ectocervical lesion

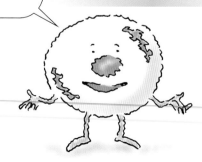

In almost all cases of cervical cancer, the histologic type is squamous cell carcinoma, which varies from well-differentiated cells to highly anaplastic spindle cells.

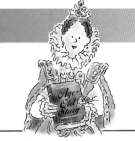

Age-old story

Age and cervical cancer

Usually, invasive carcinoma occurs in women between ages 30 and 50; it rarely occurs in those younger than age 20.

What to look for

Preinvasive disease
■ Commonly no symptoms

Early invasive disease
■ Abnormal or persistent vaginal bleeding
■ Postcoital pain and bleeding

Advanced disease
■ Pelvic pain
■ Vaginal leakage of urine and stool from a fistula
■ Anorexia, weight loss, and anemia

Risky business

Risk factors for cervical cancer

■ Frequent intercourse at a young age (younger than age 16)
■ Multiple sexual partners
■ Multiple pregnancies
■ Sexually transmitted diseases (particularly human papillomavirus)
■ Smoking

Squamous cell carcinoma in the cervix

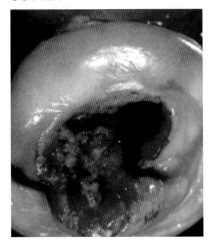

Endometrial cancer

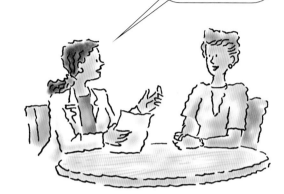

Endometrial cancer originates in the endometrium or lining of the uterus.

Also known as *uterine cancer*, endometrial cancer is the most common gynecologic cancer.

How it happens

In most cases, endometrial cancer is an adenocarcinoma that metastasizes late, usually from the endometrium to the cervix, ovaries, fallopian tubes, and other peritoneal structures. It may spread to distant organs, such as the lungs and the brain, through the blood or lymphatic system. Lymph node involvement can also occur.

Progression of endometrial cancer

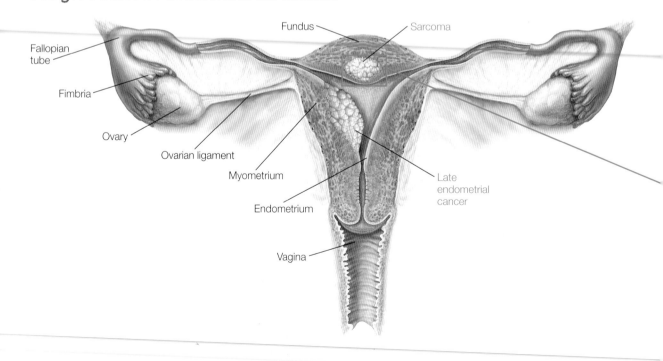

Fundus

Sarcoma

Fallopian tube

Fimbria

Ovary

Ovarian ligament

Myometrium

Endometrium

Late endometrial cancer

Vagina

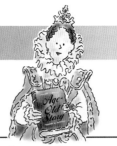

Age and endometrial cancer

Endometrial cancer commonly affects postmenopausal women between ages 50 and 60; it's uncommon between ages 30 and 40 and extremely rare before age 30. Most postmenopausal women who develop uterine cancer have a history of anovulatory menstrual cycles or other hormonal imbalance.

What to look for

■ Uterine enlargement
■ Persistent and unusual premenopausal bleeding
■ Postmenopausal bleeding
■ Pain and weight loss (advanced cancer)

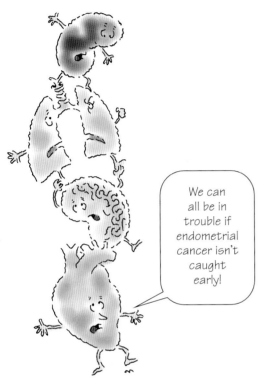

We can all be in trouble if endometrial cancer isn't caught early!

Adenocarcinoma of the endometrium

Advanced endometrial cancer

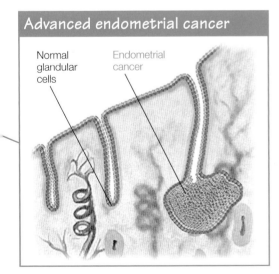

Normal glandular cells

Endometrial cancer

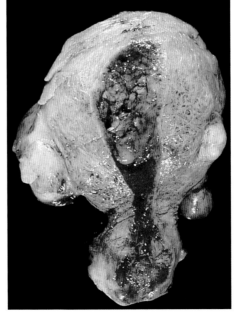

Endometriosis

Endometriosis is the presence of endometrial tissue outside the lining of the uterine cavity. Ectopic endometrial tissue is generally confined to the pelvic area, usually around the ovaries, uterovesical peritoneum, uterosacral ligaments, and the cul-de-sac, but it can appear anywhere in the body.

How it happens

The ectopic endometrial tissue responds to normal stimulation in the same way as the endometrium, but more unpredictably. The endometrial cells respond to estrogen and progesterone with proliferation and secretion. During menstruation, the ectopic tissue bleeds, which causes inflammation of the surrounding tissue. This inflammation causes fibrosis, leading to adhesions that produce pain and infertility.

Pelvic endometriosis

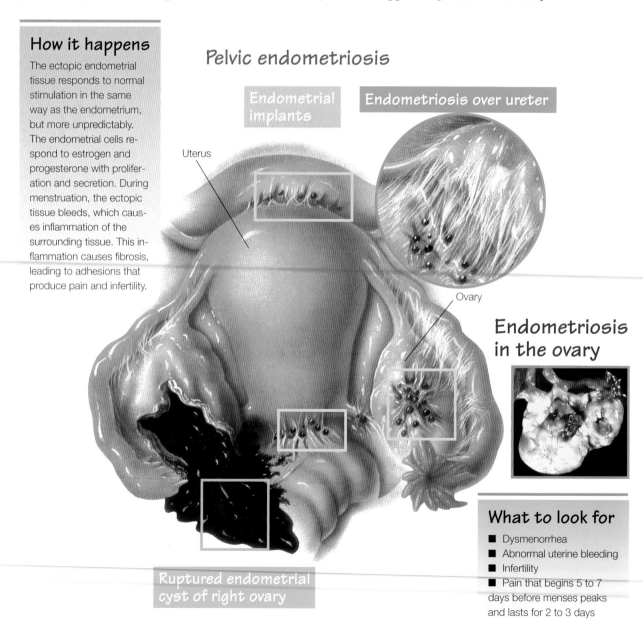

Endometrial implants

Endometriosis over ureter

Uterus

Ovary

Endometriosis in the ovary

Ruptured endometrial cyst of right ovary

What to look for

- Dysmenorrhea
- Abnormal uterine bleeding
- Infertility
- Pain that begins 5 to 7 days before menses peaks and lasts for 2 to 3 days

Common sites of endometriosis, with corresponding signs and symptoms

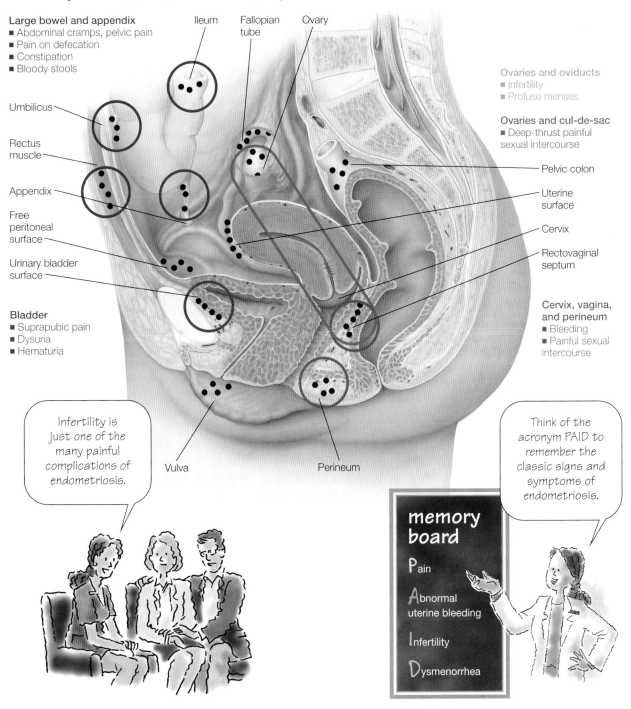

Large bowel and appendix
- Abdominal cramps, pelvic pain
- Pain on defecation
- Constipation
- Bloody stools

Umbilicus

Rectus muscle

Appendix

Free peritoneal surface

Urinary bladder surface

Bladder
- Suprapubic pain
- Dysuria
- Hematuria

Ileum

Fallopian tube

Ovary

Ovaries and oviducts
- Infertility
- Profuse menses

Ovaries and cul-de-sac
- Deep-thrust painful sexual intercourse

Pelvic colon

Uterine surface

Cervix

Rectovaginal septum

Cervix, vagina, and perineum
- Bleeding
- Painful sexual intercourse

Vulva

Perineum

Infertility is just one of the many painful complications of endometriosis.

Think of the acronym PAID to remember the classic signs and symptoms of endometriosis.

memory board

Pain

Abnormal uterine bleeding

Infertility

Dysmenorrhea

Ovarian cancer

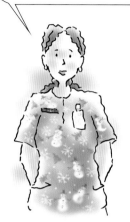

The prognosis for ovarian cancer is usually poor because ovarian tumors are difficult to diagnose and progress rapidly.

After cancers of the lung, breast, and colon, primary ovarian cancer ranks as the most common cause of cancer death among women in the United States. In women with previously treated breast cancer, metastatic ovarian cancer is more common than cancer of any other organ. The prognosis varies with the histologic type and staging of the disease.

How it happens

In ovarian cancer, primary epithelial tumors arise in the müllerian epithelium; germ cell tumors arise in the ovum; and sex cord tumors arise in the ovarian stroma. Ovarian tumors spread rapidly intraperitoneally by local extension or surface seeding and, occasionally, through the lymphatic system and the bloodstream. In most cases, extraperitoneal spread is through the diaphragm into the chest cavity, which may cause pleural effusions. Other metastasis is rare.

A closer look

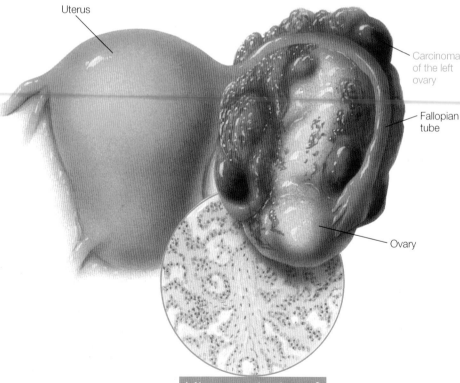

Uterus

Carcinoma of the left ovary

Fallopian tube

Ovary

Microscopic view of ovarian cancer cells

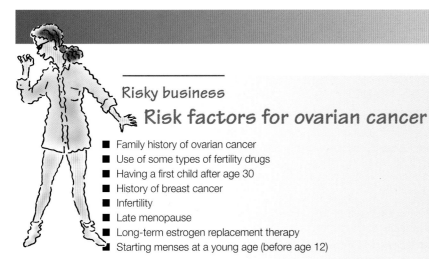

Risky business

Risk factors for ovarian cancer

- Family history of ovarian cancer
- Use of some types of fertility drugs
- Having a first child after age 30
- History of breast cancer
- Infertility
- Late menopause
- Long-term estrogen replacement therapy
- Starting menses at a young age (before age 12)

What to look for

- Vague abdominal discomfort
- Dyspepsia
- Urinary frequency
- Constipation
- Pain
- Feminizing or masculinizing effects
- Ascites
- Pleural effusions

Common metastatic sites for ovarian cancer

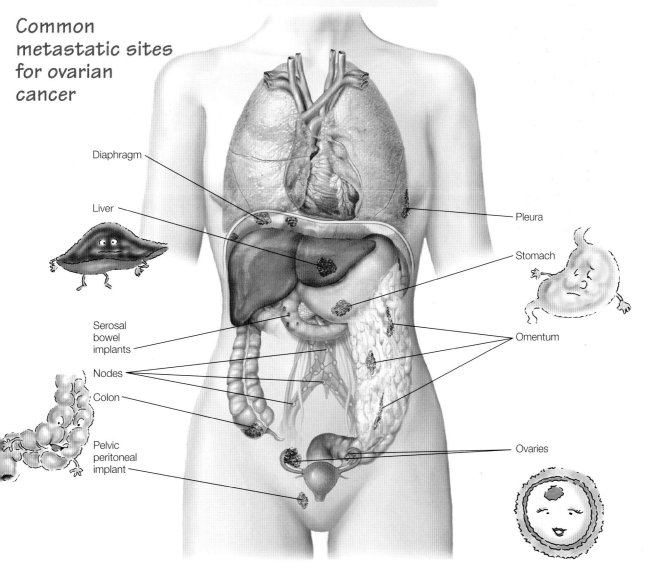

Diaphragm

Liver

Serosal bowel implants

Nodes

Colon

Pelvic peritoneal implant

Pleura

Stomach

Omentum

Ovaries

Ovarian cysts

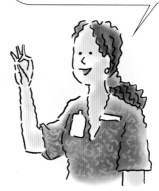

While ovarian cysts can be this small, they can cause big problems.

Ovarian cysts are usually nonneoplastic sacs on an ovary that contain fluid or semisolid material. Although these cysts are usually small and produce no symptoms, they may require thorough investigation as possible sites of malignant change.

Cysts may be single or multiple. Common physiologic ovarian cysts include follicular cysts, corpus luteum cysts, and dermoid cysts. The prognosis for nonneoplastic ovarian cysts is excellent.

How it happens

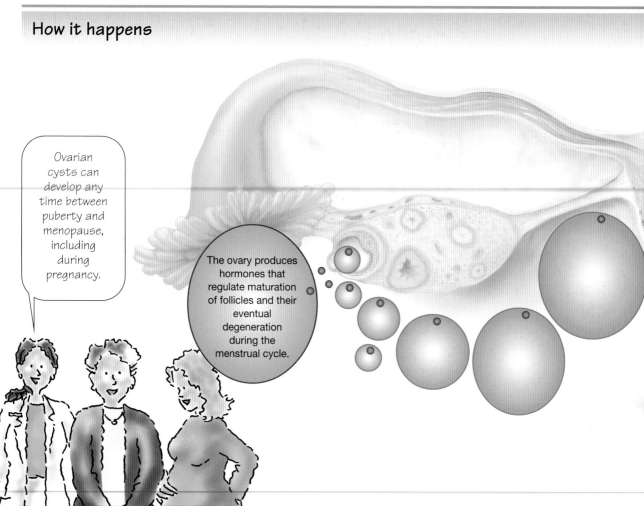

Ovarian cysts can develop any time between puberty and menopause, including during pregnancy.

The ovary produces hormones that regulate maturation of follicles and their eventual degeneration during the menstrual cycle.

The corpus luteum eventually atrophies into the corpus albicans.

The follicular cyst eventually matures to a corpus luteum after ovulation and produces progesterone until the beginning of the next menstrual cycle.

During the proliferative phase of the menstrual cycle, many follicles are released but only one reaches maturity and produces estrogen.

When follicular development into a corpus luteum doesn't occur and the follicle continues to grow, an ovarian cyst can result. Two functional ovarian cysts may develop:
• Follicular cysts
• Luteal cysts

Follicular cysts occur in the first 2 weeks of the cycle.

Corpus luteal cysts occur in the later half of the cycle.

A dermoid cyst (or cystic teratoma) begins in the ovarian cell that forms into different tissue as the egg is fertilized and develops. This type of cyst can become very large and can contain hair, teeth, bone, and cartilage. It's most common in young women and during pregnancy.

Follicular cyst

Fallopian tube

Fimbriae

Opening of the fallopian tube

Semitransparent, distended, fluid-filled cyst

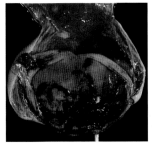

Follicular cyst of the ovary; the rupture of this thin-walled follicular cyst led to intra-abdominal hemorrhage.

Dermoid cyst

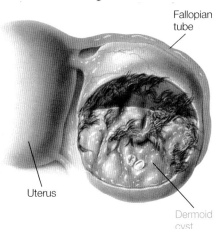

Fallopian tube

Uterus

Dermoid cyst

Prostate cancer

Prostate cancer is the most common cancer affecting men and the second cause of cancer death among men.

How it happens

About 85% of prostate cancers originate in the posterior prostate gland; the rest grow near the urethra. Adenocarcinoma is the most common form. Malignant prostatic tumors seldom result from the benign hyperplastic enlargement that commonly develops around the prostatic urethra in older men.

Slow-growing prostatic cancer rarely produces signs and symptoms until it's well advanced. Typically, when primary prostatic lesions spread beyond the prostate gland, they invade the prostatic capsule and then spread along the ejaculatory ducts in the space between the seminal vesicles or perivesicular fascia. When prostatic cancer is fatal, death usually results from widespread bone metastasis.

A closer look

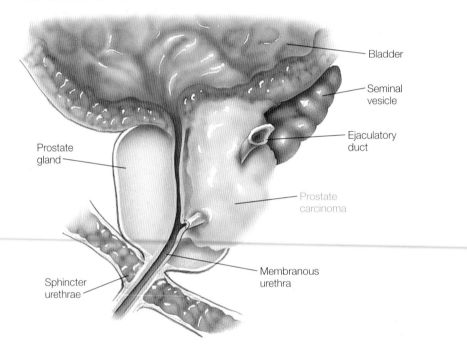

Bladder

Seminal vesicle

Ejaculatory duct

Prostate gland

Prostate carcinoma

Membranous urethra

Sphincter urethrae

What to look for

Prostate cancer seldom produces signs and symptoms until it's advanced. Signs of advanced disease are due to obstruction caused by tumor progression.
- Slow urinary stream
- Urinary hesitancy
- Incomplete bladder emptying, and dysuria

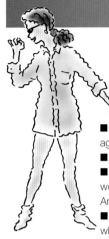

Risky business

Risk factors for prostate cancer

■ Age (more than 70% of all prostate cancer cases occur in men older than age 65)
■ Diet high in saturated fats
■ Ethnicity (Black men have the highest prostate cancer incidence in the world—more than twice that of White men. The disease is common in North America and northwestern Europe and is rare in Asia and South America.)
■ Parent or sibling with the disease. The more individuals in a family who have the disease, the greater the risk for others in the family to develop it.

Metastatic carcinoma

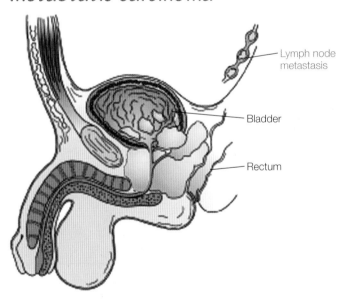

Lymph node metastasis

Bladder

Rectum

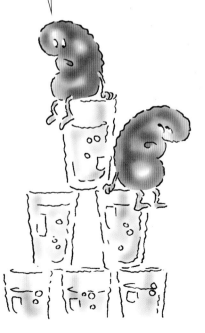

Testicular cancer

Testicular cancer accounts for less than 1% of all male cancer deaths. The prognosis depends on the cancer cell type and stage. When treated with surgery, chemotherapy, and radiation, almost all patients with localized disease survive beyond 5 years.

> With the proper treatment, most testicular cancer patients survive beyond 5 years.

How it happens

With few exceptions, testicular tumors originate from germinal cells; about 40% become seminomas. These tumors, which are characterized by uniform, undifferentiated cells, resemble primitive gonadal cells. Other tumors—non-seminomas—show various degrees of differentiation.

> Are you saying that seminoma tumors look like us primitive cells?

Typically, when testicular cancer extends beyond the testes, it spreads through the lymphatic system to the iliac, para-aortic, and mediastinal nodes. Metastases affect the lungs, liver, viscera, and bone.

Age-old story

Age and testicular cancer

Testicular cancer seldom occurs in children. Malignant testicular tumors are the most prevalent solid tumors in men ages 20 to 40.

A closer look

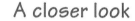

Vas deferens

Epididymis

Testis

Testicular cancer

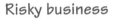

Risky business

Risk factors for testicular cancer

Although researchers don't know the immediate cause of testicular cancer, they suspect certain contributing factors.

- Cryptorchidism (undescended testis), even when surgically corrected
- History of mumps orchitis, inguinal hernia in childhood, or maternal use of diethylstilbestrol or other estrogen-progestin combinations during pregnancy
- Ethnicity (The disease is rare in men who aren't white.)

Staging testicular cancer

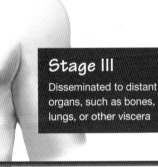

Stage III
Disseminated to distant organs, such as bones, lungs, or other viscera

Stage II
Regional nodes involved

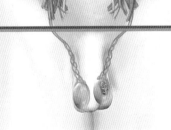

Stage I
Tumor in testis only

What to look for

Early
- Heaviness or a dragging sensation in the scrotum
- Swollen testes
- Gynecomastia
- Painless lump

Late
- Weight loss
- Cough
- Hemoptysis
- Shortness of breath
- Lethargy
- Fatigue

Uterine fibroids

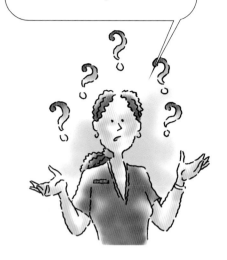

The true incidence of uterine fibroids is unknown because most women don't even know they have them.

Uterine fibroids, the most common benign tumors in women, are also known as *myomas*, *fibromyomas*, or *leiomyomas*. Uterine fibroids are tumors composed of smooth muscle and usually occur in the uterine corpus, although they may appear on the cervix or on the round or broad ligament. Uterine fibroids occur in 20% to 25% of women of reproductive age and may affect three times as many Blacks as Whites.

The tumors become malignant (leiomyosarcoma) in less than 0.1% of patients, which should serve to comfort women concerned with the possibility of a uterine malignancy in association with a fibroid.

How it happens

Leiomyomas occur from an overgrowth of smooth muscle and connective tissue in the uterus. A genetic predisposition exists. Both estrogen and progestin receptors are present in fibroids and elevated estrogen levels may cause fibroid enlargement.

During the first trimester of pregnancy, 15% to 30% of fibroids may enlarge then shrink in puerperium. Some fibroids may decrease in size during pregnancy. Fibroids shrink after menopause, but some regrowth may occur if the woman begins hormonal therapy.

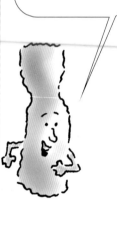

Genetically speaking, some women are predisposed to uterine fibroids.

What to look for

- Most produce no symptoms
- Abnormal bleeding
- Pain
- Pelvic pressure

A closer look

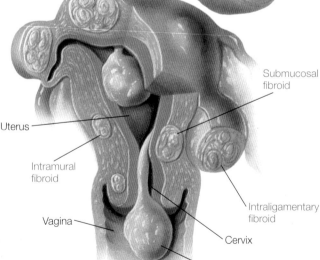

Pedunculated fibroid

Subserous fibroid

Submucosal fibroid

Uterus

Intramural fibroid

Intraligamentary fibroid

Vagina

Cervix

Pedunculated submucosal fibroid

Fibroid classification

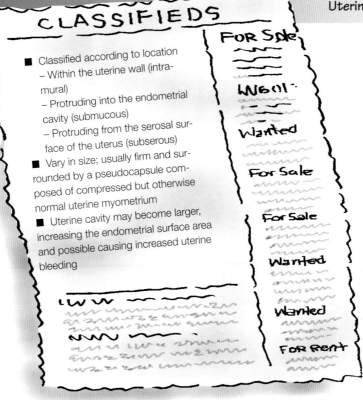

CLASSIFIEDS

■ Classified according to location
  – Within the uterine wall (intramural)
  – Protruding into the endometrial cavity (submucous)
  – Protruding from the serosal surface of the uterus (subserous)
■ Vary in size; usually firm and surrounded by a pseudocapsule composed of compressed but otherwise normal uterine myometrium
■ Uterine cavity may become larger, increasing the endometrial surface area and possible causing increased uterine bleeding

Leiomyoma of the uterus

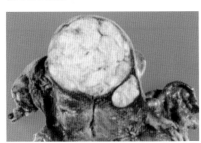

Fibroids compressing the bladder and rectum

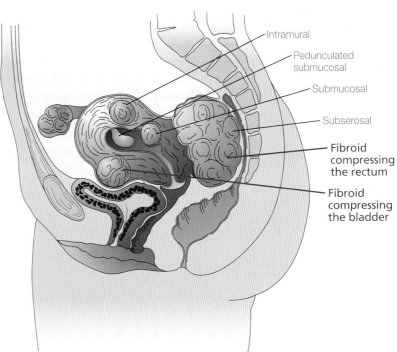

Intramural

Pedunculated submucosal

Submucosal

Subserosal

Fibroid compressing the rectum

Fibroid compressing the bladder

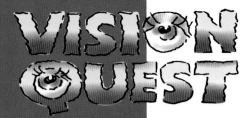

My word

Solve the word scrambles to identify terms related to reproductive disorders. Then rearrange the circled letters from those words to answer the question posed.

Question: Which reproductive disorder usually has a poor prognosis?

1. siapalrepyh _ _ _ _ ◯◯ _ _ ◯ _ _ _ _

2. oividng ◯◯ _ _ _ ◯ _

3. birofdi _ _ _ _ ◯ _ ◯ _

4. vasnievi _ ◯ _ ◯ _ _ _ _

5. llcurfoia _ _ _ _ _ _ ◯ _ _ ◯ _

6. rtaluestic _ _ _ _ _ _ ◯ _ _ _ _

Answer: _ _ _ _ _ _ _ _   _ _ _ _ _ _

Able to label?

In the illustration, label the anatomic structures involved in prostatic enlargement.

1. _____

2. _____

3. _____

4. _____

5. _____

6. _____

Selected references

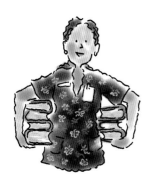

Alipour, S., et al. "Effects of Environmental Tobacco Smoke on Respiratory Symptoms and Pulmonary Function," *Inhalation Toxicology* 18(8):569-73, July 2006.

Anatomy & Physiology Made Incredibly Easy, 2nd ed. Philadelphia: Lippincott Williams & Wilkins, 2005.

Assessment Made Incredibly Easy, 3rd ed. Philadelphia: Lippincott Williams & Wilkins, 2005.

Bennett, J.S. "Vasoocclusion in Sickle Cell Anemia: Are Platelets Really Involved?" *Arteriosclerosis, Thrombosis, and Vascular Biology* 26(7):1415-16, July 2006.

Bhoola, S., and Hoskins, W.J. "Diagnosis and Management of Epithelial Ovarian Cancer," *Obstetrics & Gynecology* 107:1399-410, June 2006.

Bickley, L.S., and Szilagyi, P.G. *Bates' Guide to Physical Examination and History Taking*, 9th ed. Philadelphia: Lippincott Williams & Wilkins, 2006.

Doughty, D., et al. "Issues and Challenges in Staging of Pressure Ulcers," *Journal of Wound, Ostomy & Continence Nursing* 33(2):125-30, March-April 2006.

Gray, M., and Ratliff, C.R. "Is Hyperbaric Oxygen Therapy Effective for the Management of Chronic Wounds?" *Journal of Wound, Ostomy & Continence Nursing* 33(1):21-25, January-February 2006.

Hall, J.C. *Sauer's Manual of Skin Diseases*, 9th ed. Philadelphia: Lippincott Williams & Wilkins, 2006.

Hess, J.R., and Lawson, J.H. "The Coagulopathy of Trauma Versus Disseminated Intravascular Coagulation," *Journal of Trauma* 60(6 Suppl):S12-19, June 2006.

Kasper, D.L., et al., eds. *Harrison's Principles of Internal Medicine*, 16th ed. New York: McGraw-Hill Book Co., 2005.

Khandani, A.H., and Detterbeck, F.C. "Positron Emission Tomographic Scanning in the Diagnosis and Staging of Non-Small Cell Lung Cancer 2 cm in Size or Less," *Journal of Thoracic and Cardiovascular Surgery* 132(1):214-15, July 2006.

Porth, C.M. *Essentials of Pathophysiology: Concepts of Altered Health States*, 2nd ed. Philadelphia: Lippincott Williams & Wilkins, 2007.

Price, A.S., et al. "Impending Cardiac Tamponade: A Case Report Highlighting the Value of Bedside Echocardiography," *Journal of Emergency Medicine* 30(4):415-19, May 2006.

Rubin, E., et al. *Rubin's Pathology: Clinicopathologic Foundations of Medicine*, 4th ed. Philadelphia: Lippincott Williams & Wilkins, 2005.

Ruffolo, C., et al. "Urologic Complications in Crohn's Disease: Suspicion Criteria," *Hepatogastroenterology* 53(69):357-60, May-June 2006.

Stewart, E.A., and Morton, C.C. "The Genetics of Uterine Leiomyomata: What Clinicians Need to Know," *Obstetrics & Gynecology* 107(4): 917-21, April 2006.

Tamura, T., and Picciano, M.F. "Folate and Human Reproduction," *American Journal of Clinical Nutrition* 83(5):993-1016, May 2006.

Walsh, C., et al. "Coexisting Ovarian Malignancy in Young Women with Endometrial Cancer," *Obstetrics & Gynecology* 106(4): 693-99, October 2005.

Williams, D.T, and Liu, A.K. "Cerebral Venous Thrombosis: Hemorrhagic Stroke Requiring Acute Heparin Anticoagulation," *Journal of Emergency Medicine* 31(1):111-13, July 2006.

Credits

Chapter 1

Stages of cell division, pages 4 and 5. From Cohen, B.J., and Wood, D.L. *Memmler's The Human Body In Health and Disease*, 9th ed. Philadelphia: Lippincott Williams & Wilkins, 2000.

Chapter 2

Cardiac tamponade, page 16, bacterial endocarditis, page 24, and rheumatic valvulitis, page 41. From Rubin, E., and Farber, J.L. *Pathology*, 3rd ed. Philadelphia: Lippincott Williams & Wilkins, 1999.

Valvular heart disease, pages 37 to 41. From Porth, C.M. *Essentials of Pathophysiology: Concepts of Altered Health States*, 2nd ed. Philadelphia: Lippincott Williams & Wilkins, 2007.

Mitral valve prolapse, page 40. From Rubin, E., et al. *Rubin's Pathology: Clinicopathologic Foundations of Medicine*, 4th ed. Philadelphia: Lippincott Williams & Wilkins, 2005.

Chapter 3

Cor pulmonale, page 51. From Rubin, E., and Farber, J.L. *Pathology*, 3rd ed. Philadelphia: Lippincott Williams & Wilkins, 1999.

Adenocarcinoma of the lung, page 59, pulmonary embolus, page 67, and primary TB, page 69. From Rubin, E., et al. *Rubin's Pathology: Clinicopathologic Foundations of Medicine*, 4th ed. Philadelphia: Lippincott Williams & Wilkins, 2005.

Pneumothorax, pages 63 and 64. From Porth, C.M. *Essentials of Pathophysiology: Concepts of Altered Health States*, 2nd ed. Philadelphia: Lippincott Williams & Wilkins, 2007.

Chapter 4

Berry aneurysm, page 79, and cerebral hemorrhage, page 94. From Rubin, E., et al. *Rubin's Pathology: Clinicopathologic Foundations of Medicine*, 4th ed. Philadelphia: Lippincott Williams & Wilkins, 2005.

Chapter 5

Cirrhosis of the liver, page 101, esophageal varices photo, page 108, and necrotic liver, page 113. From Rubin, E., and Farber, J.L. *Pathology*, 3rd ed. Philadelphia: Lippincott Williams & Wilkins, 1999.

Crohn's disease, page 105, mucosal surface of the bowel in Crohn's disease, page 105, esophageal varices, pages 108 and 109, and colon with ulcerative colitis, page 117. From Rubin, E., et al. *Rubin's Pathology: Clinicopathologic Foundations of Medicine*, 4th ed. Philadelphia: Lippincott Williams & Wilkins, 2005.

Diverticulosis and diverticulitis, page 107. From National Digestive Diseases Information Clearinghouse. Clearinghouse Fact Sheet: Diverticulosis and Diverticulitis. NIH publication no. 90-1163. Washington, D.C.: U.S. Department of Health and Human Services, 1989.

Three causes of intestinal obstruction, page 114. From Smeltzer S.C., and Bare, B.G. *Brunner and Suddarth's Textbook of Medical-Surgical Nursing*, 10th ed. Philadelphia: Lippincott Williams & Wilkins, 2004.

Chapter 6

Osteoarthritis, pages 124 and 125. From Rubin, E., and Farber, J.L. *Pathology*, 3rd ed. Philadelphia: Lippincott Williams & Wilkins, 1999.

Joint changes in osteoarthritis, page 125. From Porth, C.M. *Essentials of Pathophysiology: Concepts of Altered Health States*, 2nd ed. Philadelphia: Lippincott Williams & Wilkins, 2007.

Osteosarcoma in the femur, page 133. From Rubin, E., et al. *Rubin's Pathology: Clinicopathologic Foundations of Medicine*, 4th ed. Philadelphia: Lippincott Williams & Wilkins 2005.

Chapter 8

Allergic rhinitis, page 157. From Steele, R.W. *Clinical Pediatrics* 5:656, 1966. Reprinted with permission of Sage Publications, Inc.

A closer look: ankylosing spondylitis, page 163. From Rubin, E., and Farber, J.L. *Pathology*, 4th ed. Philadelphia: Lippincott Williams & Wilkins, 2005.

A closer look: atopic dermatitis, page 165. From Goodheart, H.P. *Goodheart's Photoguide of Common Skin Disorders*, 2nd ed. Philadelphia: Lippincott Williams & Wilkins, 2003.

Chapter 9

Graves' disease, page 177, and thyroid cancer (papillary carcinoma, follicular adenoma, and medullary carcinoma), page 185. From Rubin, E., et al. *Rubin's Pathology: Clinicopathologic Foundations of Medicine*, 4th ed. Philadelphia: Lippincott Williams & Wilkins, 2005.

Chapter 10

Acute tubular necrosis, page 191, a closer look: hydronephrosis, page 195, polycystic kidney disease, page 197, a look at chronic pyelonephritis, page 199, and a look at staghorn calculi, page 201. From Rubin, E., et al. *Rubin's Pathology: Clinicopathologic Foundations of Medicine*, 4th ed. Philadelphia: Lippincott Williams & Wilkins, 2005.

Chapter 11

Adolescent facial acne, page 207. From Sauer, G.C., and Hall, J.C. *Manual of Skin Diseases*, 7th ed. Philadelphia: Lippincott-Raven Publishers, 1996.

Superficial thermal burns, page 208. David Effron, MD, 2004. Used with permission.

Burns (illustrations), pages 208 and 209. ©LifeART.

Burns (partial-thickness, full-thickness photos), page 209. From Fleisher, G.R., et al. *Atlas of Pediatric Emergency Medicine*. Philadelphia: Lippincott Williams & Wilkins, 2004.

Contact dermatitis, page 212. From Rubin, E.M. and Farber, J.L. *Pathology*, 4th ed. Philadelphia: Lippincott Williams & Wilkins, 2005.

Contact dermatitis from nickel of watch on skin, page 213. Image provided by Stedman's.

Herpes zoster, page 215. From Goodheart, H.P. *Goodheart's Photoguide of Common Skin Disorders*, 2nd ed. Philadelphia: Lippincott Williams & Wilkins, 2003.

Pressure ulcer illustrations, stages I, II, III, IV, pages 220 and 221. From Weber, J.W., and Kelley, J. *Health Assessment in Nursing*. Philadelphia: Lippincott-Raven, 1998.

Pressure ulcer photos, stages I, II, III, IV, pages 220 and 221. From Nettina, S.M. *The Lippincott Manual of Nursing Practice*, 7th ed. Philadelphia: Lippincott Williams & Wilkins, 2001.

Chapter 12

Nodular hyperplasia of the prostate, page 225, carcinoma of the breast, page 227, squamous cell carcinoma in the cervix, page 229, adenocarcinoma of the endometrium, page 231, endometriosis in the ovary, page 232, ruptured follicular cyst, page 236, metastatic carcinoma, page 239, and fibroids compressing the bladder and rectum and leimyoma of the uterus, page 243. From Rubin, E., et al. *Rubin's Pathology: Clinicopathologic Foundations of Medicine*, 4th ed. Philadelphia: Lippincott Williams & Wilkins, 2005.

We gratefully acknowledge Anatomical Chart Company for the use of selected images.

Index

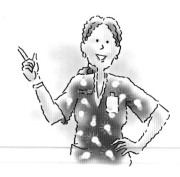